Prostate Cancer

Editors

HARSHAD R. KULKARNI
ABASS ALAVI

PET CLINICS

www.pet.theclinics.com

Consulting Editor
ABASS ALAVI

October 2022 • Volume 17 • Number 4

ELSEVIER

1600 John F. Kennedy Boulevard ● Suite 1800 ● Philadelphia, Pennsylvania, 19103-2899

http://www.pet.theclinics.com

PET CLINICS Volume 17, Number 4
October 2022 ISSN 1556-8598, ISBN-13: 978-0-323-84904-3

Editor: John Vassallo (j.vassallo@elsevier.com)
Developmental Editor: Karen Solomon

PET Clinics (ISSN 1556-8598) is published quarterly by Elsevier Inc., 360 Park Avenue South, New York, NY 10010-1710. Months of issue are January, April, July, and October. Periodicals postage paid at New York, NY, and additional mailing offices. Subscription prices per year are $262.00 (US individuals), $526.00 (US institutions), $100.00 (US students), $290.00 (Canadian individuals), $552.00 (Canadian institutions), $100.00 (Canadian students), $283.00 (foreign individuals), $552.00 (foreign institutions), and $140.00 (foreign students). To receive student and resident rate, orders must be accompanied by name of affiliated institution, date of term, and the signature of program/residency coordinator on institution letterhead. Orders will be billed at individual rate until proof of status is received. Foreign air speed delivery is included in all Clinics subscription prices. All prices are subject to change without notice. POSTMASTER: Send address changes to PET Clinics, Elsevier Health Sciences Division, Subscription Customer Service, 3251 Riverport Lane, Maryland Heights, MO 63043. **Customer Service: 1-800-654-2452 (U.S. and Canada); 314-447-8871 (outside U.S. and Canada). Fax: 314-447-8029. E-mail: journalscustomerservice-usa@elsevier.com (for print support); journalsonlinesupport-usa@elsevier.com (for online support).**

Reprints. For copies of 100 or more of articles in this publication, please contact the Commercial Reprints Department, Elsevier Inc., 360 Park Avenue South, New York, NY 10010-1710. Tel.: 212-633-3874; Fax: 212-633-3820; E-mail: reprints@elsevier.com.

PET Clinics is covered in MEDLINE/PubMed (Index Medicus).

Contributors

CONSULTING EDITOR

ABASS ALAVI, MD, MD (Hon), PhD (Hon), DSc (Hon)
Professor of Radiology and Neurology,
Director of Research Education, Division of
Nuclear Medicine, Department of Radiology,
Hospital of the University of Pennsylvania,
Perelman School of Medicine, University of
Pennsylvania, Philadelphia, Pennsylvania, USA

EDITORS

HARSHAD R. KULKARNI, MD
BAMF Health, Grand Rapids Nuclear Medicine
and Radiomolecular Theranostics, Zentralklinik
Bad Berka, Bad Berka, Germany, USA

ABASS ALAVI, MD, MD (Hon), PhD (Hon), DSc (Hon)
Professor of Radiology and Neurology,
Director of Research Education, Division of
Nuclear Medicine, Department of Radiology,
Hospital of the University of Pennsylvania,
Perelman School of Medicine, University of
Pennsylvania, Philadelphia, Pennsylvania, USA

AUTHORS

AADIL ADNAN, MD
Radiation Medicine Centre (B.A.R.C.), Tata
Memorial Hospital Annexe, Parel, Mumbai,
India; Homi Bhabha National Institute, Mumbai,
India

ABASS ALAVI, MD, MD (Hon), PhD (Hon), DSc (Hon)
Professor of Radiology and Neurology,
Director of Research Education, Division of
Nuclear Medicine, Department of Radiology,
Hospital of the University of Pennsylvania,
Perelman School of Medicine, University of
Pennsylvania, Philadelphia, Pennsylvania,
USA

SANDIP BASU, DNB
Radiation Medicine Centre (B.A.R.C.), Tata
Memorial Hospital Annexe, Parel, Mumbai, India;
Homi Bhabha National Institute, Mumbai, India

AUSTIN J. BORJA, BA
Department of Radiology, Hospital of the
University of Pennsylvania, Perelman School of
Medicine, University of Pennsylvania,
Philadelphia, Pennsylvania, USA

INDRAJA D. DEV, MD
Assistant Professor and Consultant,
Department of Nuclear Medicine and
Molecular Imaging, Tata Memorial Center,
Homi Bhabha National Institute, Mumbai, India

LIANG DONG, MD
Department of Urology, Renji Hospital,
Shanghai Jiao Tong University School of
Medicine, Shanghai, China

HEYING DUAN, MD
Research Fellow, Division of Nuclear Medicine
and Molecular Imaging, Department of
Radiology, Stanford University, Stanford,
California, USA

MICHAEL A. GORIN, MD
Milton and Carroll Petrie Department of
Urology, Icahn School of Medicine at Mount
Sinai, New York, New York, USA

POUL FLEMMING HØILUND-CARLSEN
Department of Nuclear Medicine, Odense
University Hospital, Department of Clinical
Research, University of Southern Denmark,
Denmark

CONG HU, MD
Department of Urology, Renji Hospital,
Shanghai Jiao Tong University School of
Medicine, Shanghai, China

ANDREI IAGARU, MD
Professor, Division of Nuclear Medicine and
Molecular Imaging, Department of Radiology,
Stanford University, Stanford, California,
USA

KEVIN YU JIN, MD
Department of Radiology, Hospital of the
University of Pennsylvania, Philadelphia,
Pennsylvania, USA

BENJAMIN KOA, MD
Department of Radiology, Hospital of the
University of Pennsylvania, Philadelphia,
Pennsylvania, USA

ESHA KOTHEKAR, MD
Department of Radiology, Hospital of the
University of Pennsylvania, Philadelphia,
Pennsylvania, USA

ANGIE KUANG, BS
Department of Radiology, Hospital of the
University of Pennsylvania, Philadelphia,
Pennsylvania, USA

HUI CHONG LAU, MD
Department of Medicine, Crozer-Chester
Medical Center, Upland, Pennsylvania, USA

NANCY MOHSEN, MD
Associate Professor of Clinical Radiology,
Division of Abdominal Imaging, Department of
Radiology, Hospital of the University of
Pennsylvania, Philadelphia, Pennsylvania, USA

SZE JIA NG, MD
Department of Medicine, Crozer-Chester
Medical Center, Upland, Pennsylvania, USA

PETER SANG UK PARK, BA
Department of Radiology, Hospital of the
University of Pennsylvania, Perelman School of
Medicine, University of Pennsylvania,
Philadelphia, Pennsylvania, USA

KENNETH J. PIENTA, MD
Department of Urology, The James Buchanan
Brady Urological Institute, Johns Hopkins
School of Medicine, Baltimore, Maryland, USA

MARTIN G. POMPER, MD, PhD
The Russell H. Morgan Department of
Radiology and Radiological Science, The
James Buchanan Brady Urological Institute,
Department of Urology, Johns Hopkins School
of Medicine, Baltimore, Maryland, USA

AMEYA D. PURANIK, DNB, FEBNM
Associate Professor and Consultant,
Department of Nuclear Medicine and
Molecular Imaging, Tata Memorial Center,
Homi Bhabha National Institute, Mumbai, India

WILLIAM Y. RAYNOR, MD
Department of Radiology, Hospital of the
University of Pennsylvania, Philadelphia,
Pennsylvania, USA; Department of Radiology,
Rutgers Robert Wood Johnson Medical
School, New Brunswick, New Jersey, USA

**MONA-ELISABETH REVHEIM, MD, PhD,
MHA**
Department of Radiology, Hospital of the
University of Pennsylvania, Philadelphia,
Pennsylvania, USA; Division of Radiology and
Nuclear Medicine, Oslo University Hospital,
Institute of Clinical Medicine, Faculty of
Medicine, University of Oslo, Nydalen, Oslo,
Norway; Rikshospitalet, Oslo, Norway

CHAITANYA ROJULPOTE, MD
Department of Radiology, Hospital of the
University of Pennsylvania, Philadelphia,
Pennsylvania, USA

STEVEN P. ROWE, MD, PhD
The Russell H. Morgan Department of
Radiology and Radiological Science, The
James Buchanan Brady Urological Institute,
Department of Urology, Johns Hopkins School
of Medicine, Baltimore, Maryland, USA

ALI SALAVATI, MD
The Russell H. Morgan Department of
Radiology and Radiological Science, Johns
Hopkins School of Medicine, Baltimore,
Maryland, USA

BITAL SAVIR-BARUCH, MD
Associate Professor of Radiology, Division
Chief of Nuclear Medicine, Department of
Medical Imaging, Division of Nuclear Medicine,
University of Arizona, Banner University
Medical Center-Tucson, Tucson, Arizona,
USA; Associate Professor of Radiology,
Department of Radiology, Loyola University
Chicago Stritch School of Medicine, Maywood,
Illinois, USA

DAVID M. SCHUSTER, MD, FACR
Professor (Tenure) and Director, Division of
Nuclear Medicine and Molecular Imaging, GRA
Distinguished Cancer Scientist, Department of
Radiology and Imaging Sciences, Emory
University Hospital, Atlanta, Georgia, USA

SIAVASH MEHDIZADEH SERAJ, MD
Department of Radiology, Hospital of the
University of Pennsylvania, Philadelphia,
Pennsylvania, USA

SACHI SINGHAL, MD
Department of Radiology, Hospital of the
University of Pennsylvania, Philadelphia,
Pennsylvania, USA; Department of Medicine,
Crozer-Chester Medical Center, Upland,
Pennsylvania, USA

LILJA B. SOLNES, MD, MBA
The Russell H. Morgan Department of
Radiology and Radiological Science, Johns
Hopkins School of Medicine, Baltimore,
Maryland, USA

RAHELEH TAGHVAEI, MD
Department of Radiology, Hospital of the
University of Pennsylvania, Philadelphia,
Pennsylvania, USA

RUDOLF A. WERNER, MD
The Russell H. Morgan Department of
Radiology and Radiological Science, Johns
Hopkins School of Medicine, Baltimore,
Maryland, USA; Department of Nuclear
Medicine, Wurzburg University Hospital,
Wurzburg, Germany

THOMAS J. WERNER, MSE
Department of Radiology, Hospital of the
University of Pennsylvania, Philadelphia,
Pennsylvania, USA

WEI XUE, MD, PhD
Department of Urology, Renji Hospital,
Shanghai Jiao Tong University School of
Medicine, Shanghai, China

VINCENT ZHANG, BA
Department of Radiology, Hospital of the
University of Pennsylvania, Philadelphia,
Pennsylvania, USA

Contents

Prostate cancer (PCa) is the third most common cancer diagnosed in the world. Since its first identification in 1987 and its first molecular cloning in 1993, prostate-specific membrane antigen (PSMA) has been developed as a theragnostic imaging biomarker and therapeutic agent for PCa. For metastatic castration-resistant PCa, PSMA-based PET imaging can be applied to the monitoring of disease and response assessment with PSMA-based therapeutics. This novel imaging modality is bringing new insights into diagnosis, stratification, and clinical decision-making and treatment.

Computed tomography (CT), MRI, and Ultrasound play an evolving role in prostate cancer management. Multi-parametric MRI has high sensitivity and negative predictive value in prostate cancer diagnosis, leading to increased utilization as part of an active surveillance paradigm in low-to-intermediate-risk patients, and local tumor staging in high-grade cancers. CT is modestly sensitive in staging high-grade tumors to evaluate for nodal, liver, lung, and bone metastasis, and is preferred for assessing treatment related complications. Until recently, ultrasound has been limited to a guidance modality for biopsy and treatment; however, advances in micro-ultrasound technology aim to expand its role diagnosing and managing prostate cancer.

Much of the modern growth in nuclear medicine has been driven by PET imaging of prostate-specific membrane antigen (PSMA) in men with prostate cancer. Fluorine-18 is the ideal PET radionuclide with a moderately long half-life, high positron yield, low positron energy, and cyclotron-based production. ^{18}F-DCFPyL is the first Food and Drug Administration-approved compound in this class. In this review, we cover a number of aspects of radiofluorinated PSMA PET agents, including their historical development, the early clinical trials, key multicenter registration trials, emerging clinical agents, new compounds that are entering human use, and future directions for the field.

Ameya D. Puranik and Indraja D. Dev

Imaging in prostate cancer has become increasingly important over time, as the incidence of prostate cancer has been on the rise and better screening techniques have emerged. The development of personalized systemic therapies highlights the unmet need for whole-body imaging. Prostate-specific membrane antigen (PSMA) PET, with its ease of performance and mechanism of localization to prostatic tumor cells, has now emerged as a preferred modality for diagnosis, staging, and treatment response assessment. In this context, PSMA PET can help in mapping the disease extent, both the skeletal and visceral spread, to plan targeted therapeutic approaches.

Bital Savir-Baruch and David M. Schuster

18F-Fluciclovine PET is approved for the evaluation of patients with suspected prostate cancer recurrence. 18F-Fluciclovine PET is highly specific for the localization of extraprostatic disease even with negative conventional images and low prostate-specific antigen and has been reported to influence patients' management and improve outcome. With the recent Food and Drug Administration approval of prostate-specific membrane antigen (PSMA) PET, 18F-Fluciclovine is likely to be used as an adjunct modality in patients with suspected occult local recurrence and/or negative PSMA findings.

Heying Duan and Andrei Iagaru

Molecular imaging is advancing rapidly with promising new molecular targets emerging for theragnostic, ie, imaging and treatment with the same compound, to provide targeted, personalized medicine. Gastrin-releasing peptide receptors (GRPR) are overexpressed in prostate cancer. Gallium-68 (68Ga) RM2 is a GRPR antagonist and shows high sensitivity and specificity for the detection of primary prostate cancer and recurrent disease. However, compared with the widely used 68Ga-PSMA11 and 18F-DCFPyL, a discordance in uptake pattern is seen reflecting the heterogeneity in tumor biology of prostate cancer. In this review, we present the background, current status, and future perspectives of PET imaging using 68Ga-RM2.

Benjamin Koa, William Y. Raynor, Peter Sang Uk Park, Austin J. Borja, Sachi Singhal, Angie Kuang, Vincent Zhang, Thomas J. Werner, Abass Alavi, and Mona-Elisabeth Revheim

18F-sodium fluoride (NaF) PET/computed tomography (CT) allows detection of bone metastases in patients with prostate cancer (PCa). The aim of this study was to test the feasibility of assessing global metastatic bone disease in patients with PCa by using a threshold-based PET segmentation technique. This retrospective analysis was performed in 32 patients with PCa with known bone metastases who underwent NaF-PET/CT imaging. An adaptive contrast-oriented thresholding technique was used to segment NaF avid lesions. The mean metabolic volumetric product (MVPmean), partial volume-corrected MVPmean (cMVPmean), and metabolically active volume (MAV) were calculated. Lesional values were summed within each patient to obtain the global PET disease burden. Pearson correlation analysis was used to assess the associations between global NaF-PET/CT metrics and clinical biomarkers of metastatic disease activity. Global MVPmean, cMVPmean, and MAV were significantly correlated with alkaline phosphatase (ALP) levels ($p < 0.05$). No correlation was observed between global NaF-PET/CT measures and prostate-specific antigen (PSA) levels. Global assessment is a feasible method to quantify metastatic bone disease activity in patients with PCa. Convergent validity was supported by demonstrating a significant correlation between NaF-PET/CT parameters and blood ALP levels.

Dual/multi-tracer PET-computed tomography (CT) scan has been an interesting and intriguing concept and is promising in noninvasive and overall characterization of tumor biology and heterogeneity and has scientifically augmented the practice of precision oncology. In prostate carcinoma, particularly in metastatic castration-resistant prostate carcinoma setting, dual-tracer PET-CT can be potentially useful in selecting patients for chemotherapy, androgen deprivation therapy or prostate-specific membrane antigen (PSMA)-based peptide receptor radioligand therapy either as mono-therapy or as combination therapy, ascertaining differentiation status, staging/restaging, prognostication, and predicting progression/response. PSMA PET/CT has great potential as a "rule out" test in baseline staging, while being very useful in restaging and metastatic workup.

The aim of this study was to assess coronary artery and aortic calcification in healthy controls, angina pectoris patients, and prostate cancer patients using 18F-sodium fluoride PET/computed tomography (NaF-PET/CT). A retrospective analysis compared 33 prostate cancer patients with 33 healthy subjects and 33 patients with angina pectoris. Increased target-to-background ratio (TBR) of the coronary arteries, ascending aorta, aortic arch, and descending aorta was observed in cancer patients compared to healthy controls but not compared to angina pectoris patients. These results demonstrate the feasibility of assessing vascular microcalcification with NaF-PET/CT, with significant differences in uptake according to comorbidities.

PET CLINICS

PROGRAM OBJECTIVE
The goal of the *PET Clinics* is to keep practicing radiologists and radiology residents up to date with current clinical practice in positron emission tomography by providing timely articles reviewing the state of the art in patient care.

TARGET AUDIENCE
Practicing radiologists, radiology residents, and other health care professionals who provide patient care utilizing radiologic findings.

LEARNING OBJECTIVES
Upon completion of this activity, participants will be able to:
1. Review why PET imaging can be used in the detection, staging, planning, and management of prostate cancer.
2. Discuss the advantages of using PET imaging, both traditional and novel, in accurately assessing, diagnosing, treatment planning, and predicting prostate cancer recurrences.
3. Recognize PET imaging as an effective modality in the management and treatment of prostate cancer.

ACCREDITATION
The Elsevier Office of Continuing Medical Education (EOCME) is accredited by the Accreditation Council for Continuing Medical Education (ACCME) to provide continuing medical education for physicians.

The EOCME designates this journal-based CME activity for a maximum of 9 *AMA PRA Category 1 Credit*(s)™. Physicians should claim only the credit commensurate with the extent of their participation in the activity.

All other health care professionals requesting continuing education credit for this enduring material will be issued a certificate of participation.

DISCLOSURE OF CONFLICTS OF INTEREST
The EOCME assesses conflict of interest with its instructors, faculty, planners, and other individuals who are in a position to control the content of CME activities. All relevant conflicts of interest that are identified are thoroughly vetted by EOCME for fair balance, scientific objectivity, and patient care recommendations. EOCME is committed to providing its learners with CME activities that promote improvements or quality in healthcare and not a specific proprietary business or a commercial interest.

The planning committee, staff, authors, and editors listed below have identified no financial relationships or relationships to products or devices they or their spouse/life partner have with commercial interest related to the content of this CME activity:
Aadil Adnan, MD; Abass Alavi, MD, MD (Hon), PhD (Hon), DSc (Hon); Sandip Basu, MBBS (Hons), DRM, Diplomate N.B., MNAMS; Austin J. Borja, MD; Indraja D. Dev; Liang Dong, MD; Heying Duan, MD; Poul Flemming Høilund-Carlsen, MD, PhD, DMSc, Prof (Hon); Cong Hu, MD; Andrei Iagaru, MD; Kevin Yu Jin, MD; Benjamin Koa, MD; Esha Kothekar, MD; Mohana Manoj Krishnamoorthy; Angie Kuang, MS; Harshad Kulkarni, MD; Hui Chong Lau, MD; Siavash Mehdizadeh Seraj, MD; Nancy Mohsen, MD; Sze Jia Ng, MD; Peter Sang Uk Park, MD; Ameya D. Puranik, DNB; William Y. Raynor, MD; Mona-Elisabeth Revheim, MD, PhD, MHA; Chaitanya Rojulpote, MD; Ali Salavati, MD; Sachi Singhal, MD; Lilja B. Solnes, MD, MBA; Raheleh Taghvaei, MD; Doreen Thomas-Payne, MSN, BSN, RN, PMHNP-BC; Thomas J. Werner, MSE; Rudolf A. Werner, MD; Wei Xue, MD; Vincent Zhang

The planning committee, staff, authors, and editors listed below have identified financial relationships or relationships to products or devices they or their spouse/life partner have with commercial interest related to the content of this CME activity:
Michael A. Gorin, MD: *Researcher:* Progenics Pharmaceuticals, Inc.; *Consultant*: Lantheus Pharmaceuticals, Inc., Blue Earth Diagnostics, Inc.; *Speaker*: Lantheus Pharmaceuticals, Inc.

Kenneth J. Pienta, MD: *Researcher*: Progenics Pharmaceuticals, Inc.

Martin G. Pomper, MD, PhD: *Royalties and Patent Beneficiary*: Lantheus Pharmaceuticals, Inc.; *Researcher*: Progenics Pharmaceuticals, Inc.

Steven P. Rowe, MD, PhD: *Researcher*: Progenics Pharmaceuticals, Inc.; *Consultant*: Lantheus Pharmaceuticals, Inc., Novartis AG; *Speaker*: Lantheus Pharmaceuticals, Inc.

Bital Savir-Baruch, MD: *Consultant*: Blue Earth Diagnostics, Inc., GE Healthcare; *Researcher*: Blue Earth Diagnostics, Inc.

David M. Schuster, MD, FACR: *Consultant:* AIM Specialty Health, Global Medical Solutions Taiwan, Progenics Pharmaceuticals, Inc., Syncona; *Researcher*: Advanced Accelerator Applications, Amgen Inc., Blue Earth Diagnostics, Ltd, FUJIFILM Pharmaceuticals U.S.A., Inc, Nihon MediPhysics Co, Ltd., Telix Pharmaceuticals (US) Inc.

UNAPPROVED/OFF-LABEL USE DISCLOSURE
The EOCME requires CME faculty to disclose to the participants:
1. When products or procedures being discussed are off-label, unlabelled, experimental, and/or investigational (not US Food and Drug Administration [FDA] approved); and

2. Any limitations on the information presented, such as data that are preliminary or that represent ongoing research, interim analyses, and/or unsupported opinions. Faculty may discuss information about pharmaceutical agents that is outside of FDA-approved labelling. This information is intended solely for CME and is not intended to promote off-label use of these medications. If you have any questions, contact the medical affairs department of the manufacturer for the most recent pre-scribing information.

TO ENROLL
To enroll in the *PET Clinics* Continuing Medical Education program, call customer service at 1-800-654-2452 or sign up online at http://www.theclinics.com/home/cme. The CME program is available to subscribers for an additional annual fee of USD 254.00

METHOD OF PARTICIPATION
In order to claim credit, participants must complete the following:
1. Complete enrolment as indicated above.
2. Read the activity.
3. Complete the CME Test and Evaluation. Participants must achieve a score of 70% on the test. All CME Tests and Evaluations must be completed online.

CME INQUIRIES/SPECIAL NEEDS
For all CME inquiries or special needs, please contact elsevierCME@elsevier.com.

Preface

Precision Imaging of Prostate Cancer

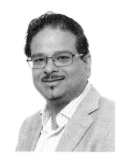
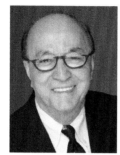

Harshad R. Kulkarni, MD   Abass Alavi, MD, PhD (Hon), DSc (Hon)

Editors

Nuclear medicine and radiomolecular theranostics has diversified into a broader field of precision oncology. PSMA PET imaging brings new insights into personalized clinical decision making and treatment of prostate cancer. Simultaneously, the role of state-of-the-art morphological imaging (computed tomography, MR imaging, and ultrasound) in the diagnosis and management of prostate cancer also continues to expand. Significant breakthroughs in prostate cancer theranostics were the FDA approval of PSMA-targeted PET imaging agents Ga-68 PSMA-11 and Pylarify, and very recently, of the radioligand therapy using Pluvicto. With the establishment of appropriate use criteria and consensus, these theranostic modalities can be further reasonably integrated into clinical trials.

PET tracers with different molecular targets and mechanisms improve the clinical management of prostate cancer. F-18 Fluciclovine, an amino acid analogue, provides a higher target-to-background signal as well as a higher specificity as compared with choline. The overexpression of gastrin-releasing peptide receptors (GRPR) in prostate cancer opens yet another radiomolecular theranostic capability, for example, in PSMA-negative metastases, using the GRPR antagonist RM-2. Ga-68 RM-2 PET imaging might further complement PSMA PET in understanding tumor biology. F-18 NaF PET represents a high-resolution imaging modality for prostate cancer, which is rather underused in the post–PSMA-PET imaging era. Indeed, further deep diving into various quantitative aspects could prove a useful supplementation to this new gold standard. F-18 FDG-PET imaging plays a decisive role in prognostication and effective personalized therapy planning, especially of a PSMA–targeted radioligand therapy.

Harshad R. Kulkarni, MD
BAMF Health
109 Michigan St NW, Suite # 700
Grand Rapids, MI 49503, USA

Abass Alavi, MD, PhD (Hon), DSc (Hon)
Division of Nuclear Medicine
Department of Radiology
University of Pennsylvania School of Medicine
Hospital of the University of Pennsylvania
3400 Spruce Street
Philadelphia, PA 19104, USA

E-mail addresses:
harshad.kulkarni@outlook.de (H.R. Kulkarni)
Abass.Alavi@pennmedicine.upenn.edu (A. Alavi)

PET Clin 17 (2022) xiii
https://doi.org/10.1016/j.cpet.2022.07.010
1556-8598/22/© 2022 Published by Elsevier Inc.

Prostate-Specific Membrane Antigen-Based PET Brings New Insights into the Management of Prostate Cancer

Cong Hu, MD[a], Liang Dong, MD[a], Wei Xue, MD, PhD[a], Kenneth J. Pienta, MD[b],*

KEYWORDS

- Prostate cancer • PET • Prostate-specific membrane antigen • Metastasis-directed therapy

KEY POINTS

- Prostate-specific membrane antigen (PSMA)-based PET provides restaging and guidance for treatment of high-risk localized prostate cancer.
- PSMA-based PET visualizes lesions and guides treatment in men with biochemical recurrence of prostate cancer.
- PSMA-based PET and radioligand therapy provide staging and an opportunity to treat metastatic prostate cancer.

INTRODUCTION

Prostate cancer (PCa) is the third most common cancer diagnosed in the world, with 1.4 million cases diagnosed and approximately 375,000 men reported dead in 2020.[1] Consequently, more accurate diagnosis, staging, and tailored treatment are needed for the management of this disease. In addition, sensitive and specific biomarkers are needed to facilitate diagnosis and treatment. Since its first identification in 1987 and the first molecular cloning in 1993, prostate-specific membrane antigen (PSMA) has been developed as a theragnostic imaging biomarker and therapeutic agent for PCa.[2–4]

Encoded by the PSMA gene, also known as the folate hydrolase 1 or glutamate carboxypeptidase 2, PSMA is a type II transmembrane glycoprotein receptor with 707 extracellular amino acids at the carboxyl terminus, 24 at the transmembrane segment, and 19 intracellular amino acids at the amino terminus.[5] This "prostate-specific" protein has also been found in other benign or malignant nonprostatic tissues and cells (salivary glands, astrocytes, melanoma, small-cell lung cancer, neovasculature of gastric and colorectal cancers, and so forth).[6–8] It is expressed in PCa cells (more than 90%), approximately 100 to 1000 times higher than that in normal prostate cells.[3,9] The increasing expression of PSMA is evident across all grades of PCa, including castration-resistant PCa (CRPCa).[10,11] The ligand of PSMA can specifically bind to the extracellular segment and trigger an endocytosis reaction, leading to the potential accumulation of radiotracers in cells, allowing the development of imaging and therapeutic antibodies or small-molecule reagents.[12] Because of the superiority in terms of binding efficiency, internalization feasibility, and plasma clearance rate, small molecule-labeled radioactive elements,

[a] Department of Urology, Renji Hospital, Shanghai Jiao Tong University School of Medicine, 160 Pujian Road, Shanghai 200127, China; [b] Department of Urology, The James Buchanan Brady Urological Institute, Johns Hopkins University School of Medicine, 600 North Wolfe Street, Baltimore, MD 21287, USA
* Corresponding author.
E-mail address: kpienta1@jhmi.edu

PET Clin 17 (2022) 555–564
https://doi.org/10.1016/j.cpet.2022.07.001
1556-8598/22/© 2022 Elsevier Inc. All rights reserved.

such as ^{68}Ga, ^{18}F, ^{111}In, and ^{177}Lu are leading the trend for imaging and therapeutic use.[13]

The combination of PET and computed tomography (CT) or PET and magnetic resonance (MR) and PSMA highlights its advantages in achieving a more accurate diagnosis with improved sensitivity and specificity.[14–23] PSMA-based PET not only successfully converts foci not clinically evident under conventional imaging (CI, eg, CT, MRI, and bone scintigraphy) to visible lesions in different settings but also has the potential to alter the treatment and management of PCa patients.[24–26] With the approval of two PSMA imaging agents (^{68}Ga-PSMA-11 and ^{18}F-DCFPyL) in the past 2 years by the US Food and Drug Administration (FDA), access to novel imaging is expanding rapidly in the United States.[27,28] Furthermore, the National Comprehensive Cancer Network (NCCN)'s adoption of PSMA-based PET in updated guidelines, the appropriate use criteria (AUC)[29] for PSMA-based PET, and the consensus on the guidance of better integration into clinical trials[30] support the more widespread application of this imaging modality in a more standardized manner. Compared with CI, the cost-effectiveness of ^{68}Ga-PSMA PET/MRI for men with biochemical recurrence demonstrates positive trends in health system costs and years of life (survival) over 10 years.[31] PSMA-based PET will impact the management of PCa in several ways.

Providing Restaging and Guidance for Treatment in High-Risk Localized Prostate Cancer

In PCa patients, PSMA-based PET has distinct advantages over CI modalities (CT, MRI, bone scan, PET scan) [20,30] (Fig. 1). PSMA-based PET imaging techniques are applicable to detect the location of PCa lesions in primary and recurrent cancer.[32,33] When a physician stratifies a patient into a certain risk group according to his clinicopathological characteristics, "high risk" refers to the risk of recurrence or disease metastasis. In a high-risk patient, for example, whose primary tumor was removed and a distal bone metastasis was found several years after radical prostatectomy (RP), it is likely that the bone lesion had already been present at the time of surgery but undetectable by CI. If the bone lesion was detectable by PSMA-based PET at the time of surgery, this could guide a change in management.

A recent prospective study enrolled 30 patients with diagnosed primary PCa (histologically proven intermediate or high risk) to explore the diagnostic performance of ^{18}F-DCFPyL-PET/CT (^{18}F-labeled PSMA ligand) in foci detection within the gland. The findings show that per-patient detection (93%) and localization in clinically significant PCa (Gleason score $\geq 3 + 4 = 7$) are accurate. It directly showed a high consistency between imaging findings and actual sites.[34,35] With the impressive detection rate, it appears that PSMA-PET can be utilized for TNM staging and the following treatment decision-making. The utility of PSMA-based PET among unfavorable intermediate-to-very-high-risk PCa patients validated by histopathology and preoperative efficacy in N-staging has been verified.[36] Evaluation of lymph node (LN) metastasis is vitally important to determine whether extended pelvic lymph node dissection (ePLND) should be applied during RP. Ferraro and colleagues found that ^{68}Ga-PSMA PET/MRI accurately detected pelvic suspicious LNs with a sensitivity of 58% and a high specificity of 98%, indicating its potential to select optimal candidates for ePLND in intermediate-to-high-risk PCa.[37] The most common site of distant metastases of prostate adenocarcinoma is bone (Fig. 2), and PSMA-based PET has high sensitivity and specificity for lesion identification, contributing to M-staging.[38] Pomykala and colleagues found that 49 out of 70 patients (70%) underwent restaging of M1 disease, demonstrating that PSMA-PET could identify bone metastases of PCa in a timely and comprehensive manner even in the presence of low serum PSA levels.[39]

In another study, 14% (20 of 148) of patients had their therapy changed from curative to palliative-intent treatment with first-line PSMA-based PET. Seven percent of them (11 of 148) received a change in radiotherapy planning, and another 7% (11 of 148) received an altered surgical plan.[26] These studies demonstrate that PSMA-PET identifies PCa that has escaped the prostate, altering treatment plans for patients. PSMA-PET is especially valuable as it detects additional nodal involvement, altering surgical, radiation, and systemic treatment decisions.[40] Overall, as high-risk localized PCa with potential involvement of LNs or distant metastases is accurately diagnosed, the resulting stage migration may translate into better outcomes for patients.

Providing Restaging and Guidance for Treatment in Men with a Biochemical Recurrence

According to the European Association of Urology (EAU) and the American Urologic Association, biochemical recurrence (BCR) is defined as two consecutive confirmations of serum PSA greater than 0.2 ng/mL after RP or an increase in PSA level

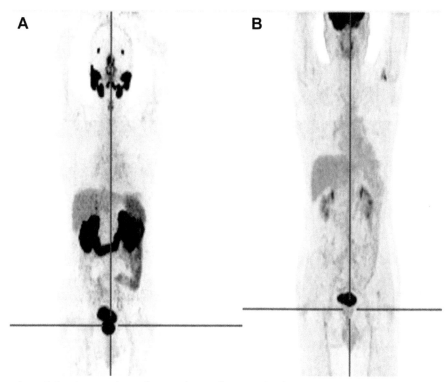

Fig. 1. Overview of visual comparison of PET and CT with two radiopharmaceuticals in the same patient. (A) ^{68}Ga-PSMA (B) ^{18}F-FDG. The prostate is marked out.

by 2.0 ng/mL or more above the nadir after radical radiotherapy, with concurrent negative CI.[41,42] Approximately 70% of patients who received either RP or radiotherapy to treat their primary tumors will be cured, while the remaining 30% will develop BCR. In approximately 40% of these men, treatment will fail, and it will eventually progress to metastatic disease.[43,44] Identifying disease at the BCR stage offers the possibility of potential curative salvage therapy. However, due to the limited sensitivity of CI (CT scan, MRI, and whole-body technetium bone scans) at low PSA levels, the current treatments for BCR are not precisely directed.[45,46] According to pooled data, ^{68}Ga-PSMA-11 shows an improved detection rate of metastases in the BCR group,[22] especially at low pre-PET PSA levels of less than 0.2 ng/mL (33%) and 0.2 to 0.5 ng/mL (45%).[47] When PET-CT imaging is considered for patients with BCR after RP with a low PSA of less than 2.0 ng/mL to make subsequent treatment management decisions, PSMA-based ligands demonstrate improved disease detection.[48] Fabio and colleagues demonstrated a high detection rate (over 70%) in BCR patients with PSMA-based PET/CT when PSA was below 1 ng/mL. In addition, no differences were found among PSMA-based radiotracers evaluated by prostate-specific antigen

doubling time (PSADT) or prostate-specific antigen velocity, and their superiority over "old" radiotracers, such as choline-based ligands was observed.[49] In addition to PSA level, other predictors, such as PSADT, can be used to predict scan positivity and disease location.[23,50] Dong and colleagues explored the best candidates for PSMA PET/CT scans based on the EAU BCR risk categories.[51] When compared with low-risk (PSADT >12 months and GS < 8 after RP), high-risk BCR patients (patients with PSADT ≤12 months or GS ≥ 8 after RP) had a higher positive rate.[52]

Considering the factors involved in the improved detection rate in the setting of BCR, PSMA-based PET makes invisible foci under CI visible. Accurate foci localization will define the best candidates who are likely to benefit from subsequent therapy, such as salvage or metastasis-directed therapy (MDT). However, the benefit of MDT remains unclear. Some studies have demonstrated a reduction in the risk of further progression and delayed systematic treatment but others have not shown a benefit.[53–55] In one study, PCa patients received RP and underwent MDT [salvage lymph node dissection (sLND)] for nodal recurrence detected by PSMA-based PET.[53] Nearly 33% of patients died 10 years after surgery at a long-term

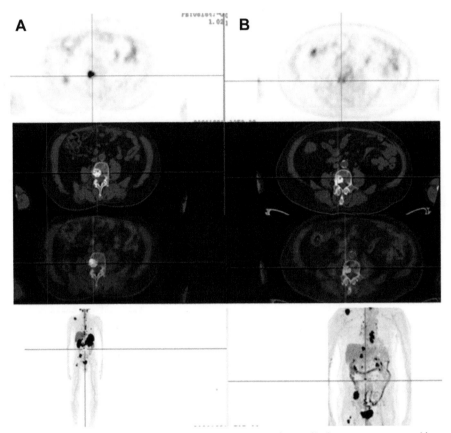

Fig. 2. A 75-year-old man with systemic multiple bone metastases after radical prostatectomy and hormone therapy (A) ^{68}Ga-PSMA. (B) ^{18}F-FDG. Relatively better display of metastases in the vertebral body with PSMA-based PET.

assessment, and only a minority of them benefited from the additional procedure. sLND alone was not recommended for patients with only nodal recurrence. Clinical trials and longer follow-up are needed to determine if identifying metastatic disease earlier and subsequent early therapy—whether MDT or systemic—will alter patient outcomes.

Providing Staging and Guidance for Treatment in Metastatic Prostate Cancer

The expression of PSMA throughout the stages of PCa offers the possibility of staging, following treatment response, and treatment with PSMA-radioligand therapy (RLP) in patients with metastatic disease. It has been shown that androgen-deprivation therapy leads to increased PSMA expression in PCa, and high PSMA uptake and high administered radionuclide dose were associated with a higher chance of treatment response.[20,56–58] With the failure of conventional therapies, such as chemotherapy or novel hormone therapy (ie, abiraterone, enzalutamide) in

advanced refractory stages, PSMA-based radioactive molecules are providing new treatment options for PCa. Since its introduction worldwide,[59] its demonstrated advantage of efficacy with good biosafety over conventional treatments has been increasingly accepted clinically.[60] Accordingly, PSMA-based PET is evolving in terms of determining the optimal candidates and evaluating and monitoring their response to treatment.[61–63] RLP represented by ^{177}Lu-PSMA-617 prolonged both imaging-based progression-free survival (median, 8.7 months) and overall survival (median, 15.3 months) when combined with standard care compared with the latter alone (3.4 and 11.3 months, respectively).[64] The VISION trial demonstrated favorable results of RLP facilitating the application of ^{177}Lu-PSMA-617.[65]

The LuPSMA trial[66], a single-center, single-arm, phase 2 study, administered up to four cycles of intravenous ^{177}Lu-PSMA-617 (with a 6-week interval) to 30 progressed metastatic CRPC patients after the confirmation of high PSMA expression according to PSMA-based PET/CT. PSA response was assessed as the primary endpoint, with

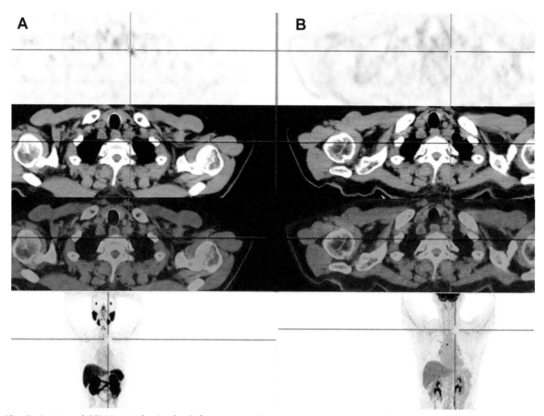

Fig. 3. Increased PSMA uptake in the left upper mediastinal nerve root area after hormone therapy for PCa is considered a high probability of physiologic uptake. (*A*) ^{68}Ga-PSMA. (*B*) ^{18}F-FDG.

evaluated imaging response and quality of life as the additional primary endpoints. However, 57% of patients [95% confidence interval (CI) 37–75) demonstrated a PSA decline of 50% or more. Another trial compared [1][77]Lu-PSMA-617 with cabazitaxel (considered to be the next appropriate standard of care) in the same patient group, the result of which demonstrated a higher PSA response and fewer grade 3 or 4 adverse events.[67] A 50% PSA decline was achieved in 32 of 50 patients (64%; 95% CI, 50%–77%), and 44% of patients achieved an approximate decrease of more than 80%. The median follow-up time was 31.4 months, and the median overall survival time was 13.3 months (95% CI, 10.5–18.7). Patients with at least a 50% decrease in PSA demonstrated a longer survival time of 18.4 months (95% CI, 13.8–23.8). Moreover, improved quality of life was observed with [1][77]Lu-PSMA-617 therapy. The Brief Pain Inventory severity and interference scores decreased at all time points, and the pain scale on the EORTC QLQ-C30 improved accordingly.[68] Based on targeted therapy with these radionuclide drugs, PSMA-PET will be increasingly valued as an indicator of lesion evaluation and as a means of monitoring treatment response.

Early diagnosis and treatment monitoring is feasible for metastatic CRPC,[69] and(RLTs) are promising. It should be noted, however, that in the setting of neuroendocrine PCa (NEPC), its efficacy remains to be explored due to the lack of PSMA embedded in the cell membrane.[70]

A Few Caveats for Utilization of Prostate-Specific Membrane Antigen-Based PET in Clinical Use

PSMA is expressed on PCa cell membranes and correlates to some extent with the degree of disease progression.[58,71] However, PSMA exists partially in both benign and malignant tissues, which can lead to false positive results.[8,9,11] The PSMA uptake is observed in other tissues and organs, such as the lacrimal glands, parotid glands, kidneys, liver, and urinary tract,[72] which increases the chance of misinterpreting some of the imaging results. Studies are trying to reduce the binding of the nonspecific residues to reduce the background interference.[73] Therefore, PSMA-PET imaging must be interpreted carefully. For example, uptake by sympathetic ganglia may be misinterpreted in localized PCa as metastases to

Table 1
New insights into different functional perspectives of prostate-specific membrane antigen-based imaging with prostate cancer

Dimensions	Superiority	Limitations
Detection	Primary prostate cancer: Accurate localization of intraprostatic foci, lymph nodes, and bone with high sensitivity and specificity Biochemical recurrence: Making the foci previously invisible visible	Certain minor lesions can be missed
Staging	More accurate staging for the assessment of the disease	Challenges in primary staging in low-risk prostate cancer
Treatment	Tailoring treatment based on prostate-specific membrane antigen ligands and PET imaging modality	The availability of the therapy needs to be extended.
Relevant changes	Adjusted therapy according to the PET results	Adequate data and uniform standard are needed

nonregional LNs.[74,75] A case of PSMA uptake by neural tissue is shown in **Fig. 3**. In addition, in some PCa, including NEPC (<10%),[11] PSMA-based PET imaging results are inherently negative.[76] Another issue in this regard is accessibility. The accessibility of PSMA-based radiopharmaceuticals needs to be improved both for imaging and therapy applications. For example, the use of ^{68}Ga-PSMA-11 was approved by the FDA in late 2020,[28] but the relatively high cost and the lack of radiotracer limit the general availability of the technology. Furthermore, the interpretation of PSMA imaging on patient outcomes will be hampered in the near term by lead time bias. Although lesions are detected earlier with PSMA-PET, and it appears that early treatment prolongs overall survival time, the time from the onset of the disease to death may not change. The better clinical outcomes of the participation of PSMA-based PET imaging modalities in the management of PCa patients need to be demonstrated with more access to high-quality research and standardized clinical trial guidance.[30] Some brief but important points are listed in Table 1 (**Table 1**).

SUMMARY

Based on the properties of PSMA, the novel PSMA-based PET imaging modality provides new insights into the management of PCa patients. Compared with CI techniques, PSMA-PET has unique advantages in different scenarios. First, the high sensitivity and specificity in patients with primary and recurrent PCa allow for a much higher detection rate within the prostate, LNs, bone, and other sites, facilitating diagnostic biopsies with accuracy. Second, PSMA-PET can facilitate the staging of PCa patients and change

the management of patients, contributing to further treatment. Third, PSMA ligand and PSMA-based PET present new directions in terms of targeting and monitoring of the disease, offering a new modality for the tailored treatment of PCa. In the light of our discussion so far, we are confident that PSMA-PET will revolutionize the diagnosis and treatment of PCa.

CLINICS CARE POINTS

- PSMA-based PET imaging modality provides new insights into the management of PCa patients.
- PSMA has high sensitivity and specificity in patients with primary and recurrent PCa.
- P SMA-PET can facilitate the staging of PCa patients and change the management of patients.

DISCLOSURE

The authors have nothing to disclose.

REFERENCES

1. Siegel RL, Miller KD, Fuchs HE, et al. Cancer statistics, 2022. CA Cancer J Clin 2022;72(1):7–33.
2. Israeli RS, Powell CT, Fair WR, et al. Molecular cloning of a complementary DNA encoding a prostate-specific membrane antigen. Cancer Res 1993; 53(2):227–30.

3. Horoszewicz JS, Kawinski E, Murphy GP. Mono-
clonal antibodies to a new antigenic marker in
epithelial prostatic cells and serum of prostatic cancer patients. Anticancer Res 1987;7(5b):927–35.

4. Ristau BT, O'Keefe DS, Bacich DJ. The prostate-
specific membrane antigen: lessons and current
clinical implications from 20 years of research. Urol
Oncol 2014;32(3):272–9.

5. Leek J, Lench N, Maraj B, et al. Prostate-specific
membrane antigen: evidence for the existence of a
second related human gene. Br J Cancer 1995;
72(3):583–8.

6. Robinson MB, Blakely RD, Couto R, et al. Hydrolysis
of the brain dipeptide N-acetyl-L-aspartyl-L-gluta-
mate. Identification and characterization of a novel
N-acetylated alpha-linked acidic dipeptidase activity from rat brain. J Biol Chem 1987;262(30):
14498–506.

7. Nimmagadda S, Pullambhatla M, Chen Y, et al. Low-
level endogenous PSMA expression in nonprostatic
tumor xenografts is sufficient for in vivo tumor targeting and imaging. J Nucl Med 2018;59(3):486–93.

8. Haffner MC, Kronberger IE, Ross JS, et al. Prostate-
specific membrane antigen expression in the neovasculature of gastric and colorectal cancers. Hum
Pathol 2009;40(12):1754–61.

9. Kinoshita Y, Kuratsukuri K, Landas S, et al. Expression of prostate-specific membrane antigen in
normal and malignant human tissues. World J Surg
2006;30(4):628–36.

10. Bostwick DG, Pacelli A, Blute M, et al. Prostate specific membrane antigen expression in prostatic intra-
epithelial neoplasia and adenocarcinoma: a study of
184 cases. Cancer 1998;82(11):2256–61.

11. Silver DA, Pellicer I, Fair WR, et al. Prostate-specific
membrane antigen expression in normal and malignant human tissues. Clin Cancer Res 1997;3(1):81–5.

12. Ghosh A, Heston WDW. Tumor target prostate specific membrane antigen (PSMA) and its regulation
in prostate cancer. J Cell Biochem 2004;91(3):
528–39.

13. Hofman MS, Hicks RJ, Maurer T, et al. Prostate-specific membrane antigen PET: clinical utility in prostate cancer, normal patterns, pearls, and pitfalls.
Radiographics Jan-feb 2018;38(1):200–17.

14. Wang R, Shen G, Yang R, et al. 68)Ga-PSMA PET/
MRI for the diagnosis of primary and biochemically
recurrent prostate cancer: a meta-analysis. Eur J
Radiol 2020;130:109131.

15. Rowe SP, Macura KJ, Ciarallo A, et al. Comparison
of prostate-specific membrane antigen-based 18F-
DCFBC PET/CT to conventional imaging modalities
for detection of hormone-naïve and castration-
resistant metastatic prostate cancer. J Nucl Med
2016;57(1):46–53.

16. Rowe SP, Macura KJ, Mena E, et al. PSMA-based
[(18)F]DCFPyL PET/CT is superior to conventional

imaging for lesion detection in patients with metastatic prostate cancer. Mol Imaging Biol 2016;18(3):
411–9.

17. Hu X, Wu Y, Yang P, et al. Performance of 68Ga-
labeled prostate-specific membrane antigen ligand
positron emission tomography/computed tomography in the diagnosis of primary prostate cancer: a
systematic review and meta-analysis. Int Braz J
Urol 2021;47. https://doi.org/10.1590/s1677-5538.
Ibju.2020.0986.

18. Evangelista L, Zattoni F, Cassarino G, et al. PET/MRI
in prostate cancer: a systematic review and meta-
analysis. Eur J Nucl Med Mol Imaging 2021;48(3):
859–73.

19. Jansen BHE, Bodar YJL, Zwezerijnen GJC, et al.
Pelvic lymph-node staging with (18)F-DCFPyL PET/
CT prior to extended pelvic lymph-node dissection
in primary prostate cancer - the SALT trial. Eur J
Nucl Med Mol Imaging 2021;48(2):509–20.

20. Vlachostergios PJ, Niaz MJ, Skafida M, et al. Imaging expression of prostate-specific membrane antigen and response to PSMA-targeted β-emitting
radionuclide therapies in metastatic castration-
resistant prostate cancer. Prostate 2021;81(5):
279–85.

21. Kopp J, Kopp D, Bernhardt E, et al. 68Ga-PSMA
PET/CT based primary staging and histological correlation after extended pelvic lymph node dissection
at radical prostatectomy. World J Urol 2020;38(12):
3085–90.

22. Martinez J, Subramanian K, Margolis D, et al. 68Ga-
PSMA-HBED-CC PET/MRI is superior to multiparametric magnetic resonance imaging in men with
biochemical recurrent prostate cancer: a prospective single-institutional study. Transl Oncol 2022;
15(1):101242.

23. Xue AL, Kalapara AA, Ballok ZE, et al. 68)Ga-Pros-
tate-Specific membrane antigen positron emission
tomography maximum standardized uptake value
as a predictor of gleason pattern 4 and pathological
upgrading in intermediate-risk prostate cancer.
J Urol 2022;207(2):341–9.

24. Sonni I, Eiber M, Fendler WP, et al. Impact of (68)Ga-
PSMA-11 PET/CT on staging and management of
prostate cancer patients in various clinical settings:
a prospective single-center study. J Nucl Med
2020;61(8):1153–60.

25. Abufaraj M, Grubmüller B, Zeitlinger M, et al. Prospective evaluation of the performance of [(68)Ga]
Ga-PSMA-11 PET/CT(MRI) for lymph node staging
in patients undergoing superextended salvage
lymph node dissection after radical prostatectomy.
Eur J Nucl Med Mol Imaging * 2019;46(10):2169–77.

26. Hofman MS, Lawrentschuk N, Francis RJ, et al.
Prostate-specific membrane antigen PET-CT in patients with high-risk prostate cancer before
curative-intent surgery or radiotherapy (proPSMA):

a prospective, randomised, multicentre study. Lancet 2020;395(10231):1208–16.

27. FDA approves a second PSMA targeting agent for PET imaging in men with prostate cancer. BJU Int 2021;128(2):127–30.

28. FDA Approves First PSMA-Targeted PET Drug. J Nucl Med 2021;62(2):11n.

29. Jadvar H, Calais J, Fanti S, et al. Appropriate use criteria for prostate-specific membrane antigen PET imaging. J Nucl Med 2022;63(1):59–68.

30. Schöder H, Hope TA, Knopp M, et al. Considerations on integrating prostate-specific membrane antigen positron emission tomography imaging into clinical prostate cancer trials by national clinical trials Network Cooperative groups. J Clin Oncol 2022;Jco2102440. https://doi.org/10.1200/jco.21.02440.

31. Gordon LG, Elliott TM, Joshi A, et al. Exploratory cost-effectiveness analysis of (68)Gallium-PSMA PET/MRI-based imaging in patients with biochemical recurrence of prostate cancer. Clin Exp Metastas 2020;37(2):305–12.

32. Xiang M, Ma TM, Savjani R, et al. Performance of a prostate-specific membrane antigen positron emission tomography/computed tomography-derived risk-stratification tool for high-risk and very high-risk prostate cancer. JAMA Netw Open 2021;4(12):e2138550.

33. Klingenberg S, Jochumsen MR, Ulhøi BP, et al. 68)Ga-PSMA PET/CT for primary lymph node and distant metastasis NM staging of high-risk prostate cancer. J Nucl Med 2021;62(2):214–20.

34. Bodar YJL, Jansen BHE, van der Voorn JP, et al. Detection of prostate cancer with (18)F-DCFPyL PET/CT compared to final histopathology of radical prostatectomy specimens: is PSMA-targeted biopsy feasible? The DeTeCT trial. World J Urol 2021;39(7):2439–46.

35. Hope TA, Goodman JZ, Allen IE, et al. Metaanalysis of (68)Ga-PSMA-11 PET accuracy for the detection of prostate cancer validated by histopathology. J Nucl Med 2019;60(6):786–93.

36. Langbein T, Wang H, Rauscher I, et al. Utility of (18)F-rhPSMA-7.3 positron emission tomography for imaging of primary prostate cancer and pre-operative efficacy in N-staging of unfavorable intermediate to very high-risk patients validated by histopathology. J Nucl Med 2022. https://doi.org/10.2967/jnumed.121.263440.

37. Ferraro DA, Muehlematter UJ, Garcia Schüler HI, et al. 68)Ga-PSMA-11 PET has the potential to improve patient selection for extended pelvic lymph node dissection in intermediate to high-risk prostate cancer. Eur J Nucl Med Mol Imaging 2020;47(1):147–59.

38. Zhou J, Gou Z, Wu R, et al. Comparison of PSMA-PET/CT, choline-PET/CT, NaF-PET/CT, MRI, and bone scintigraphy in the diagnosis of bone metastases in patients with prostate cancer: a systematic review and meta-analysis. Skeletal Radiol 2019;48(12):1915–24.

39. Pomykala KL, Czernin J, Grogan TR, et al. Total-body 68Ga-PSMA-11 PET/CT for bone metastasis detection in prostate cancer patients: potential impact on bone scan guidelines. J Nucl Med 2020;61(3):405–11.

40. Afaq A, Payne H, Davda R, et al. A Phase II, Open-label study to assess safety and management change using (68)Ga-THP PSMA PET/CT in patients with high risk primary prostate cancer or biochemical recurrence after radical treatment: the PRONOUNCED study. J Nucl Med 2021;62(12):1727–34.

41. Thompson IM, Valicenti RK, Albertsen P, et al. Adjuvant and salvage radiotherapy after prostatectomy: AUA/ASTRO guideline. J Urol 2013;190(2):441–9.

42. Cornford P, Bellmunt J, Bolla M, et al. EAU-ESTRO-SIOG guidelines on prostate cancer. Part II: treatment of relapsing, metastatic, and castration-resistant prostate cancer. Eur Urol 2017;71(4):630–42.

43. Han M, Partin AW, Zahurak M, et al. Biochemical (prostate specific antigen) recurrence probability following radical prostatectomy for clinically localized prostate cancer. J Urol 2003;169(2):517–23.

44. van der Toom EE, Axelrod HD, de la Rosette JJ, et al. Prostate-specific markers to identify rare prostate cancer cells in liquid biopsies. Nat Rev Urol 2019;16(1):7–22.

45. Song H, Harrison C, Duan H, et al. Prospective evaluation of (18)F-DCFPyL PET/CT in biochemically recurrent prostate cancer in an Academic center: a focus on disease localization and changes in management. J Nucl Med 2020;61(4):546–51.

46. Rowe SP, Campbell SP, Mana-Ay M, et al. Prospective evaluation of PSMA-targeted (18)F-DCFPyL PET/CT in men with biochemical failure after radical prostatectomy for prostate cancer. J Nucl Med 2020;61(1):58–61.

47. Perera M, Papa N, Roberts M, et al. Gallium-68 prostate-specific membrane antigen positron emission tomography in advanced prostate cancer-updated diagnostic utility, sensitivity, specificity, and distribution of prostate-specific membrane antigen-avid lesions: a systematic review and meta-analysis. Eur Urol 2020;77(4):403–17.

48. Calais J, Ceci F, Eiber M, et al. F-18-fluciclovine PET-CT and Ga-68-PSMA-11 PET-CT in patients with early biochemical recurrence after prostatectomy: a prospective, single-centre, single-arm, comparative imaging trial. Lancet Oncol 2019;20(9):1286–94.

49. Crocerossa F, Marchioni M, Novara G, et al. Detection rate of prostate specific membrane antigen tracers for positron emission tomography/computerized tomography in prostate cancer biochemical

recurrence: a systematic review and Network meta-analysis. J Urol 2021;205(2):356–69.

50. Mena E, Rowe SP, Shih JH, et al. Predictors of (18)F-DCFPyL-PET/CT positivity in patients with biochemical recurrence of prostate cancer after local therapy. J Nucl Med 2021. https://doi.org/10.2967/jnumed.121.262347.

51. Van den Broeck T, van den Bergh RCN, Briers E, et al. Biochemical recurrence in prostate cancer: the European association of Urology prostate cancer guidelines panel recommendations. Eur Urol Focus 2020;6(2):231–4.

52. Dong L, Su Y, Zhu Y, et al. The European association of Urology biochemical recurrence risk groups predict findings on PSMA PET in patients with biochemically recurrent prostate cancer after radical prostatectomy. J Nucl Med 2021. https://doi.org/10.2967/jnumed.121.262411.

53. Bravi CA, Fossati N, Gandaglia G, et al. Long-term outcomes of salvage lymph node dissection for nodal recurrence of prostate cancer after radical prostatectomy: not as good as previously thought. Eur Urol 2020;78(5):661–9.

54. Grubmüller B, Baltzer P, D'Andrea D, et al. 68)Ga-PSMA 11 ligand PET imaging in patients with biochemical recurrence after radical prostatectomy - diagnostic performance and impact on therapeutic decision-making. Eur J Nucl Med Mol Imaging 2018; 45(2):235–42.

55. Morris MJ, Carroll PR, Saperstein L, et al. Impact of PSMA-targeted imaging with 18F-DCFPyL-PET/CT on clinical management of patients (pts) with biochemically recurrent (BCR) prostate cancer (PCa): results from a phase III, prospective, multicenter study (CONDOR). J Clin Oncol 2020;38(15).

56. Wright GL Jr, Grob BM, Haley C, et al. Upregulation of prostate-specific membrane antigen after androgen-deprivation therapy. Urology 1996;48(2): 326–34.

57. Sweat SD, Pacelli A, Murphy GP, et al. Prostate-specific membrane antigen expression is greatest in prostate adenocarcinoma and lymph node metastases. Urology 1998;52(4):637–40.

58. Evans MJ, Smith-Jones PM, Wongvipat J, et al. Noninvasive measurement of androgen receptor signaling with a positron-emitting radiopharmaceutical that targets prostate-specific membrane antigen. Proc Natl Acad Sci U S A 2011;108(23): 9578–82.

59. Kratochwil C, Giesel FL, Eder M, et al. [^{177}Lu]Lutetium-labelled PSMA ligand-induced remission in a patient with metastatic prostate cancer. Eur J Nucl Med Mol Imaging 2015;42(6):987–8.

60. Zang J, Liu QX, Sui HM, et al. Lu-177-EB-PSMA radioligand therapy with escalating doses in patients with metastatic castration-resistant prostate cancer. J Nucl Med 2020;61.

61. Heinzel A, Boghos D, Mottaghy FM, et al. 68)Ga-PSMA PET/CT for monitoring response to (177)Lu-PSMA-617 radioligand therapy in patients with metastatic castration-resistant prostate cancer. Eur J Nucl Med Mol Imaging 2019;46(5):1054–62.

62. Giesel FL, Hadaschik B, Cardinale J, et al. F-18 labelled PSMA-1007: biodistribution, radiation dosimetry and histopathological validation of tumor lesions in prostate cancer patients. Eur J Nucl Med Mol Imaging 2017;44(4):678–88.

63. Pollard JH, Raman C, Zakharia Y, et al. Quantitative test-retest measurement of Ga-68-PSMA-HBED-CC in tumor and normal tissue. J Nucl Med 2020; 61(8):1145–52.

64. Sartor O, de Bono J, Chi KN, et al. Lutetium-177-PSMA-617 for metastatic castration-resistant prostate cancer. N Engl J Med 2021;385(12):1091–103.

65. Jadvar H. The VISION forward: recognition and implication of PSMA-/FDG+ mCRPC. J Nucl Med 2021. https://doi.org/10.2967/jnumed.121.263274.

66. Hofman MS, Violet J, Hicks RJ, et al. [Lu-177]-PSMA-617 radionuclide treatment in patients with metastatic castration-resistant prostate cancer (LuPSMA trial): a single-centre, single-arm, phase 2 study. Lancet Oncol 2018;19(6):825–33.

67. Hofman MS, Emmett L, Sandhu S, et al. [(177)Lu]Lu-PSMA-617 versus cabazitaxel in patients with metastatic castration-resistant prostate cancer (TheraP): a randomised, open-label, phase 2 trial. Lancet 2021;397(10276):797–804.

68. Violet J, Sandhu S, Iravani A, et al. Long-term follow-up and outcomes of retreatment in an expanded 50-patient single-center phase II prospective trial of (177)Lu-PSMA-617 theranostics in metastatic castration-resistant prostate cancer. J Nucl Med 2020;61(6):857–65.

69. Weber M, Kurek C, Barbato F, et al. PSMA-ligand PET for early castration-resistant prostate cancer: a retrospective single-center study. J Nucl Med 2021;62(1):88–91.

70. Pouliot F, Beauregard JM, Saad F, et al. The Triple-Tracer strategy against Metastatic PrOstate cancer (3TMPO) study protocol. BJU Int 2021. https://doi.org/10.1111/bju.15621.

71. Hofman MS, Iravani A. Gallium-68 prostate-specific membrane antigen PET imaging. PET Clin 2017; 12(2):219–34.

72. Noto B, Büther F, Auf der Springe K, et al. Impact of PET acquisition durations on image quality and lesion detectability in whole-body (68)Ga-PSMA PET-MRI. EJNMMI Res 2017;7(1):12.

73. Harsini S, Saprunoff H, Alden T, et al. The effects of monosodium glutamate on PSMA radiotracer uptake in men with recurrent prostate cancer: a prospective, randomized, double-blind, placebo-controlled intraindividual imaging study. J Nucl Med 2021; 62(1):81–7.

74. Sheikhbahaei S, Werner RA, Solnes LB, et al. Prostate-specific membrane antigen (PSMA)-Targeted PET imaging of prostate cancer: an update on important pitfalls. Semin Nucl Med 2019;49(4):255–70.

75. Rischpler C, Beck TI, Okamoto S, et al. 68)Ga-PSMA-HBED-CC uptake in Cervical, Celiac, and sacral ganglia as an important pitfall in prostate cancer PET imaging. J Nucl Med 2018;59(9):1406–11.

76. Usmani S, Ahmed N, Marafi F, et al. Molecular imaging in neuroendocrine differentiation of prostate cancer: 68Ga-PSMA versus 68Ga-DOTA NOC PET-CT. Clin Nucl Med 2017;42(5):410–3.

Role of MRI, Ultrasound, and Computed Tomography in the Management of Prostate Cancer

Nancy Mohsen, MD

KEYWORDS

- Prostate cancer • Local staging • CT • Multi-parametric MRI • Active surveillance
- Biochemical tumor recurrence • Micro-ultrasound • Metastasis

KEY POINTS

MRI role in Gleason Grade Groups 1, 2, and 3.

- Identify additional cancers or suspicious lesions that may have been missed by transrectal ultrasound (TRUS) biopsy and target lesions for a follow-up MR–US fusion biopsy.
- Confirm finding of low-volume tumor at TRUS that could be misinterpreted because of sampling error.
- Evaluate for T3 disease (extracapsular extension and seminal vesicle invasion), which may elevate the patient risk group.
- If the patient undertakes an active surveillance approach, then MRI can play a role along with prostate-specific antigen, before periodic TRUS-guided biopsies, to increase sensitivity for new or increasing grade tumor.

After a diagnosis of prostate cancer has been confirmed, anatomic imaging techniques including ultrasound, computed tomography (CT), and multi-parametric MRI (mp-MRI) continue to play evolving roles in management.[1] There are five basic roles, including initial staging of intermediate- and high-risk prostate cancer,[1–8] assessment of complications after definitive treatment of cancers,[9] evaluation for local tumor recurrence in patients with treated high-risk cancer who have biochemical recurrence or progression on androgen deprivation therapy,[5] active surveillance of patients with very low and low risk tumors,[7] and image guidance for targeting of lesions for biopsy in the setting of suspected recurrence or suspected conversion of low-grade to higher-grade tumors.[10]

In the management of diagnosed prostate cancer, there are three general pathways for management determined by tumor stage, risk group, and shared decision-making with the patient. These include active surveillance, localized therapy (radiation, surgery, high-intensity focused ultrasound, and cryotherapy), and systemic therapy (androgen deprivation therapy and chemotherapy/immunotherapy).

mp-MRI of the prostate/pelvis is used in tumor staging of intermediate-to-high-risk prostate cancer mainly to assess for pelvic lymphadenopathy and extracapsular extension, whereas whole-body MRI, where available, is used to evaluate for distant metastasis.[5] A benefit of CT is the lack of ionizing radiation. mp-MRI also plays an increasing role in the active surveillance of very

No commercial or financial conflicts of interest.

Division of Abdominal Imaging, Department of Radiology, Hospital of the University of Pennsylvania, 1 Silverstein Suite 130, 3400 Spruce Street, Philadelphia, PA 19104, USA

E-mail address: nancy.mohsen@pennmedicine.upenn.edu

PET Clin 17 (2022) 565–583
https://doi.org/10.1016/j.cpet.2022.07.002

low/low risk prostate cancer.[7] The high negative predictive value of mp-MRI can be leveraged for the selection of active surveillance candidates. In patients already on active surveillance, it can also be used to detect higher risk disease.[7] However, up to 20% of Prostate Imaging Reporting and Data System (PIRADS) 3 lesions will show clinically significant (Gleason 4) disease indicating that MRI surveillance cannot replace biopsy in an active surveillance protocol.[7]

CT is used in the staging of intermediate to high-risk prostate cancer for pelvic lymphadenopathy and distant metastasis (including liver, lung, and bone),[11,12] whereas in current practice ultrasound has been predominantly useful as a tool for guidance during prostate biopsy either alone or fused with MRI. Conventional trans-rectal/trans-perineal ultrasound has not proven to be reliable in the differentiation of clinically significant prostate nodules[1] with sensitivity and specificity ranging from 40% to 50% on multiple studies.

Several recent studies show the promise of emerging micro-ultrasound techniques in the identification of clinically significant prostate cancer using a portable ultrasound system in the urologist's office, suggesting these techniques have the potential to play a larger role in the management of prostate cancer in the near future. One meta-analysis of 11 studies shows similar sensitivity and positive predictive value of prostate micro-ultrasound when compared with multi-parametric MRI in the detection of cancer.[13,14] The research in this field is rapidly evolving, however, this has yet to be validated via large multicenter trials.

PROSTATE CANCER RISK GROUP ASSESSMENT

Not all diagnosed prostate cancer is clinically significant or in need of treatment.[15–18] Treatments for prostate cancer are often associated with complications that significantly impact quality of life, such as urinary and erectile dysfunction.[9,18] Furthermore, many localized prostate cancers found to be of low risk will never progress to metastasis, become symptomatic during the patient's lifetime, or result in death.[15,17,18]

Current management strategies and guidelines favor less aggressive approaches in patients with cancers that are at low risk to progress in order to prevent morbidity related to overtreatment.[17,18] Determining which patients are low to very low risk and who would benefit from either watchful waiting or an active surveillance approach is critical.

Risk group is determined by a combination of prostate-specific antigen (PSA, Gleason score/grade group, tumor volume, and clinical stage based on digital rectal examination and imaging.[16,18] Additional parameters such as biochemical markers can be used in challenging cases as a problem-solving tool. The role of anatomic imaging, specifically mp-MRI, in the decision tree continues to be more precisely defined as new data emerges.

GLEASON SCORE AND GLEASON PROGNOSTIC GRADE GROUP

After transrectal ultrasound (TRUS) biopsy, the pathologist assigns a Gleason score to each specimen, reflecting histopathologic grade based on the glandular pattern. Gleason score is reported as 2 numbers and their sum. The first number indicates the most common type of glandular formation seen within each biopsy sample on a scale of 1 to 5, and the second number is the second most common pattern in the sample, followed by the sum of the 2 (ie, $4 + 5 = 9$). A score of 1 would indicate a normal glandular pattern whereas a score of 5 would indicate complete replacement by abnormal cells/tissue. Generally, Gleason score sums of 6 and above are consistent with clinically significant prostate cancer.

Because a low-grade prostate cancer has a Gleason score of up to 6, and the scale ranges from 2 to 10, there was a developing need to prevent the false perception among patients that a Gleason 6 is an intermediate-grade cancer, and to differentiate between Gleason $3 + 4$ and $4 + 3$ cancers that have differing prognoses.[19] This is most important when guiding patients toward less aggressive treatment approaches such as active surveillance. Reporting of Gleason Grade Groups developed from this need, with groups from 1 to 5, based on Gleason sum scores, with group 1 indicating the lowest risk of prostate cancer (Gleason $3 + 3 = 6$ and less) and Gleason grade group 5 the highest. The grade group is intended to give clinicians and their patients a clear sense of tumor histopathologic grade and highlights the differentiation in grade between Gleason $3 + 4 = 7$ (Gleason grade group 2) and $4 + 3 = 7$ (Gleason grade group 3) (**Table 1**).

PROSTATE-SPECIFIC ANTIGEN

PSA scores less than 10 ng/mL are associated with low-risk disease, 10 to 20 ng/mL with intermediate-risk disease, and greater than 20 with high-risk disease.[1]

CLINICAL T STAGE

The clinical T stage for risk group assessment is determined by rectal examination to assess for palpable mass, and imaging.[16,18] Non-palpable

Table 1
Gleason prognostic grade group

Gleason Score	Gleason Prognostic Grade Group
3 + 3 = 6	1
3 + 4 = 7	2
4 + 3 = 7	3
4 + 4 = 8	4
4 + 5, 5 + 4 = 9, or 5 + 5 = 10	5

Data from Pierorazio PM, Walsh PC, Partin AW, Epstein JI. Prognostic Gleason grade grouping: data based on the modified Gleason scoring system. BJU Int. 2013 May;111(5):753–760.

mass is clinical stage T1. Palpable lesions, or those visible on ultrasound or MRI, are clinical stage T2. This stage can be further subdivided based on whether the tumor involves less than 50% of one side of the prostate (T2a), greater than 50% of one side of the prostate (T2b), or involves both sides of the prostate (T2c). Lesions that have directly extended outside the prostate into seminal vesicle or adjacent fat are T3, whereas those that have extended into adjacent organs including the bladder, urethral sphincter, or rectum are T4.

Combining these factors with the number of biopsy specimens containing prostate cancer/overall tumor volume determines the risk group (**Table 2**).

There are multiple risk group assessment scales used throughout the world for the determination of the risk of recurrence of prostate cancer to help guide management. The most widely used classification system in the United States has been the D'Amico system, which delineates three major risk groups: low, intermediate, and high.[20] These can each be further subdivided into additional groups using the AUA/ASTRO/SUO consensus guidelines and the recently developed British Cambridge Prognostic Group (CPG) classification. The D'Amico low-and intermediate-risk groups are subdivided into two additional groups, very low/low risk, and intermediate-risk groups are divided into favorable and unfavorable, via the AUA/ASTRO/SUO guidelines. They chose no further subdivision of high risk given that it would not affect management. The CPG subdivides the D'Amico intermediate and high-risk categories into groups 2 to 5[16,18] (see **Table 1**).

RISK GROUPS

Low-risk prostate cancer is non-palpable, Gleason grade group 1 (Gleason score 6 or less),

with PSA less than 10. Most of these patients can safely undergo an active surveillance program. In some patients who are uncomfortable with the active surveillance approach, or have risk factors for clinical progression (perineural invasion, African American Race, family history or genetic predisposition to metastatic or lethal prostate cancer, body mass index (BMI) > 35 kg/m, or PSA density >0.15 ng/mL) definitive therapy with radical prostatectomy or radiation therapy is recommended.[16] Imaging staging for metastasis is not recommended for low-risk patients unless patient is symptomatic. If a patient with low to intermediate risk prostate cancer has a life expectancy of less than 5 years, a watchful waiting program is favored that recognizes that treatment-related morbidity is greater than the risk that progressive disease will result in symptoms or death.

Intermediate-risk patients have Gleason grade group 2 or 3 (Gleason score 7), or PSA of 10 to 20 ng/mL, or a palpable lesion on digital rectal examination. A consensus paper by the AUA/ASTRO/SUO in 2017 further subdivides this risk group into favorable and unfavorable categories. This subdivision is based on the differential prognostic risk that has been found between Gleason Grade groups 2 and 3, with Grade group 2 having a favorable prognosis in the absence of a second feature. Favorable intermediate-risk patients in some instances can be followed with active surveillance. Favorable intermediate-risk patients are Gleason 3 + 4 (Gleason grade group 2), *or* have a PSA 10 to 20 ng/mL, whereas unfavorable intermediate-risk patients have Gleason grade group 2 lesions *and* PSA 10 to 20 or Gleason grade group 3 (Gleason 4 + 3). In patients with unfavorable intermediate-risk prostate cancer, the American Urologic Association recommends imaging with multiparametric MRI for local staging, bone scan, and CT to evaluate for nodal and distant metastasis.[1,16]

High-risk disease is characterized by a Gleason 8 to 10 (Grade group 4 or 5), or PSA greater than 20 ng/mL, or greater than clinical stage T2c. Patients with the localized high-risk disease will benefit from definitive treatment with prostatectomy with or without external beam radiation therapy and subsequent maintenance androgen deprivation therapy. Alternatively, radiation therapy with androgen deprivation therapy can be used for these patients in lieu of surgery with similar long-term outcomes. For these patients, CT for the evaluation of distant metastasis and bone scan is recommended as well as multiparametric MRI to assess for local tumor spread.[1,16]

Table 2
Prostate cancer Risk Group Assessment table

D'amico Risk Group 1998	Parameters	Cambridge Prognostic Group (CPG) 2021	Parameters	AUA/ASTRO/SUO 2017	Parameters
Low risk	• Gleason Grade Group 1 (score 6 or less) and • PSA <10 ng/mL and • Clinical T1 - T2a	1	• Gleason score 6 or less (Grade Group 1) and • PSA <10 ng/mL and • Clinical T1–T2a	VERY LOW RISK	No more than one-third positive random core biopsies (this excludes targeted biopsy specimens) No core >50% involvement Gleason grade group 1 (Gleason score <6) PSA density <0.15 ng/mL/cc
				LOW RISK	PSA < 10 and Gleason grade group 1 and clinical stage T1–T2A
Intermediate risk	• Gleason score 7 OR • PSA 10–20 ng/mL OR • Stage T2b–c	2	• Gleason score 3 + 4 = 7 (Grade Group 2) OR • PSA 10–20 ng/mL AND Stages T1–T2	INTERMEDIATE FAVORABLE	Gleason grade group 2 and PSA < 10 or Gleason grade group 1 and PSA 10–20 ng/mL
		3	• Gleason score 3 + 4 = 7 (Grade Group 2) and PSA 10–20 ng/mL or stages T1–T2 OR • Gleason score 4 + 3 = 7 (Grade Group 3) AND stages T1–T2	INTERMEDIATE UNFAVORABLE	Grade group 2 and PSA 10–20 ng/ml or clinical stage T2b–c Or Grade Group 3 with PSA < 20 ng/mL
High risk	Gleason score 8–10 (Grade Group 4 or 5) OR PSA >20 ng/mL OR Stage ≥ T2c	4	One of: • Gleason score 8 (Grade Group 4) OR • PSA > 20 ng/mL or • Stage T3	HIGH RISK	Gleason score 8–10 (Grade Group 4 or 5) OR PSA >20 ng/mL OR Stage ≥ T3
		5	Any combination of: • Gleason score 8–10 (Gleason grade groups 4–5) • PSA > 20 ng/mL or • Stage T3 or stage T4		

ROLE OF MRI

Prostate MRI has dramatically evolved over the past 20 years in the diagnosis of prostate cancer with the advent of standardized imaging protocols using mp-MRI and standardized reporting using the PIRADS latest version 2.1.[21] Widespread adoption of the PIRADS risk assessment scale, which grades the likelihood a prostate lesion is clinically significant prostate cancer (Gleason 7 or above) on a scale of 1 to 5. This is based on objective imaging features using three parameters, which include diffusion-weighted signal, T2 signal and morphology, and dynamic contrast enhancement. PIRADS 3 lesions are "intermediate suspicion" whereas PIRADS 4 and 5 are "suspicious" and "highly suspicious" for clinically significant prostate cancer. Studies have shown a sensitivity ranging from 74% to 80% and specificity of 80% to 93%, a positive predictive value of 90.0%, and a negative predictive value of 89.6% in identifying Gleason 7 and above prostate lesions.[21,22] Although MRI for the initial diagnosis of prostate cancer is outside of the scope of this discussion, it is important to understand the power of this tool in identifying clinically significant prostate cancer as it pertains to patient risk stratification and the growing importance of MRI in the active surveillance of patients with low-to-intermediate grade prostate cancer.

Of all the current imaging modalities, MRI provides the highest anatomic resolution both within the prostate delineating the zonal anatomy, and outside the prostate differentiating between the prostate and surrounding tissue.[21,23,24] The latter feature proves to be important in the evaluation of local tumor spread (**Fig. 1**).

MRI IN LOW-TO-INTERMEDIATE GRADE TUMORS

In patients, where low-to-intermediate-grade or low-volume prostate adenocarcinoma is identified at TRUS-guided biopsy, MRI is of benefit. In these patients an active surveillance approach is often strongly considered. The use of MRI in this setting is two-fold. The first goal is to identify additional suspicious lesions (PIRADS 3 or above) within the prostatic tissue that was not sampled at initial biopsy, that could have a higher Gleason grade or T-stage. For the biopsy proven low-grade or intermediate grade prostate adenocarcinoma, MRI is used to confirm the overall low tumor volume and low T stage of biopsy proven lesions, in patients whenan active surveillance approach is being considered. If MRI identifies suspicious lesions that were not previously sampled, then typically a second ultrasound-guided MR-fusion targeted biopsy is performed on the lesions identified at MRI (**Fig. 2**).

In 2017 the Prostate MR Imaging Study (PROMIS), a multicenter paired cohort study performed in the United Kingdom, sought to determine whether adding MRI before TRUS biopsy in patients with elevated serum PSA could allow MRI to be used as a triage test to avoid unnecessary biopsy and potential complications while improving diagnostic accuracy. The sensitivity and specificity of mp-MRI and TRUS biopsy for Gleason 7 and above cancer were each compared against trans-perineal template mapping biopsies in patients with PSA up to 15 ng/mL.[1,23] PROMIS showed significantly superior sensitivity (88%) and negative predictive value (76%) of mp-MRI in diagnosing any Gleason 7 and above prostate cancer compared with TRUS biopsy (sensitivity 48%, negative predictive value (NPV) 63%). If clinically significant prostate cancer is defined as Gleason 4 + 3 and above, the sensitivity and negative predictive value of MRI improved to 93% and 89%, respectively,[23] whereas TRUS biopsy, sensitivity, and NPV are 48% and 74%, respectively.[23] These findings suggested that MRI used as a triage test before biopsy could allow 27% of men at risk to avoid unnecessary biopsy and could reduce the diagnosis of clinically insignificant cancer by 5%. Based on this data, the authors concluded that if TRUS biopsies were directed by mp-MRI findings, an additional 18% of clinically significant cancer cases could be diagnosed.[23]

Also of importance in this study was the finding that 17 of 576 men had negative mp-MRI but clinically significant prostate cancer. All of these undetected cases were Gleason 3 + 4 or less. In contrast, of the 119 significant cancers missed by TRUS, 13 were Gleason 4 + 3, whereas the remainder were Gleason 3 + 4 or less. As a result of these findings in the active surveillance population, it has become clear that mp-MRI or TRUS biopsy cannot be used in isolation. Patients must still undergo some combination of surveillance periodic TRUS biopsies, mp-MRI, and PSA. Moreover, the utility of mp-MRI in the targeting of lesions before biopsy has become increasingly evident.

In active surveillance patients, increasing tumor size and decreasing ADC has been associated with increased tumor grade.[21,23]

MRI in Intermediate-to-High Grade Prostate Cancer

In patients with intermediate-to-high grade tumors at biopsy, mp-MRI provides an important information regarding local staging. Because of

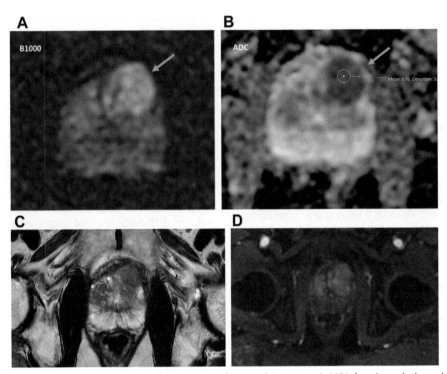

Fig. 1. (*A, B*) Diffusion weighted b1000 and ADC images from multiparametric MRI showing a lesion with marked signal abnormality with left anterior prostate with associated gross extracapsular extension. (*C, D*) T2-weighted and early post-contrast images from multiparametric MRI showing a lesion with low T2 signal and ill-defined margins within the left anterior prostate with associated anterior gross extracapsular extension and early contrast enhancement measuring greater than 1.5 cm consistent with a PIRADS 5 lesion. ADC, apparent diffusion coefficient.

the inherently superior tissue contrast of MRI, extracapsular extension, seminal vesicle invasion, bladder and rectal invasion are characterized with a greater degree of confidence and accuracy by MRI, compared with CT. Nonetheless, there continues to be room for improvement in the MRI diagnosis of local T3 disease (extension to seminal vesicles and peri-prostatic fat). Several studies have shown that patients with extraprostatic extension (EPE) are at increased risk for positive margins at surgery, metastasis, and biochemical recurrence. Therefore, accurate characterization of extracapsular extension before the determination of treatment pathway is important.[25]

A meta-analysis by Maarten de Rooij[2], evaluating the accuracy of MRI imaging for local staging of prostate cancer, revealed a low sensitivity of 61% and specificity of 88% in identifying T3 disease with slightly higher sensitivities in patients where 3T MRI (rather than 1.5 or 1.0 T) and high-resolution T2-weighted images were used. Interestingly, they also showed that in studies with high field strength 3T magnets, endorectal coil use provided no improvement in detection and actually showed lower rates of EPE detection.

Some improvement in detection was seen when an endorectal coil was used with 1.5 T or less field strength magnets. These findings were not significantly different for detecting seminal vesicle invasion or extracapsular extension (**Fig. 3**).

Several features have been suggested as increasing the likelihood of T3 disease. Rosenkrantz and colleagues[25] studied the length of capsular contact by tumor as an independent predictor of extracapsular extension and found 6 mm for focal EPE and 10 mm for non-focal EPE on T2-weighted imaging as threshold values to improve the detection and inter-observer agreement for EPE. Mehralivand and colleagues[26] proposed a grading system for assessing the risk of EPE. They proposed 3 levels of risk based on the presence of curvilinear contact length of tumor to capsule or capsular bulge or irregularity (24.3% risk), the presence of both of these features (38.2% risk), or frank breach of the prostatic capsule (66.1% risk).

In evaluating for bone metastasis, whole-body MRI is more sensitive and specific than CT or bone scan. In combination with multiparametric MRI of the prostate, whole-body MRI may allow for single modality prostate cancer staging.[5]

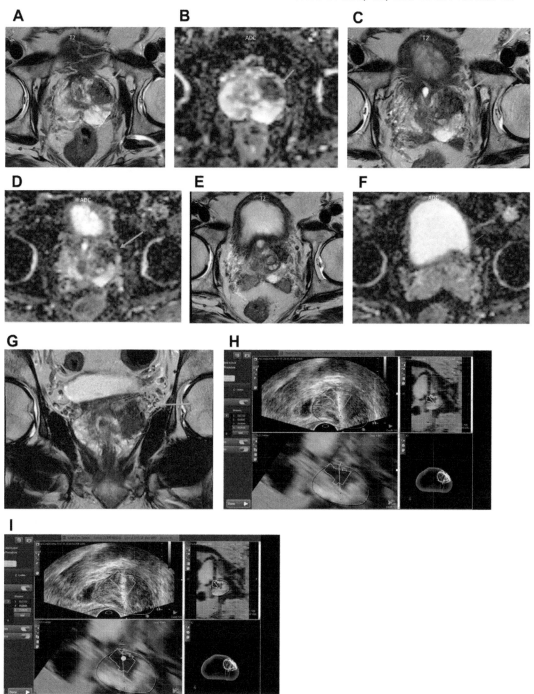

Fig. 2. (*A, B*) A 69–year-old man with PSA elevated to 18. Multiparametric MRI showing T2-weighted image on the left and ADC map on the right displaying a large left anterior base lesion greater than 1.5 cm correlating to a PIRADS 5 lesion. (*C, D*) A 69-year-old man with PSA elevated to 18. Multiparametric MRI showing T2-weighted image on the left and ADC map on the right displaying a large left anterior base lesion greater than 1.5 cm correlating to a PIRADS 5 lesion. There is a long curvilinear area of capsular contact, capsular bulging and irregularity consistent with extraprostatic extension (blue arrow). (*E, F*) A 69-year-old man with PSA elevated to 18. Multiparametric MRI showing T2-weighted image on the left and ADC map on the right displaying a large left anterior base lesion greater than 1.5 cm correlating to a PIRADS 5 lesion. Signal abnormality extending to the left bladder neck suspicious for invasion. (*G*) T2-weighted coronal sequence shows gross extraprostatic tumor extension to better advantage (*blue arrow*) and again possible bladder neck involvement (*green arrow*). (*H, I*) Images from ultrasound MRI fusion biopsy. Ultrasound image is superimposed on a volumetric reconstruction of the prostate for tumor targeting for fusion biopsy. Samples identified Gleason 8 tumor in the target lesion. ([*A-E*] *Courtesy of* Exact Imaging, Markham, Ontario).

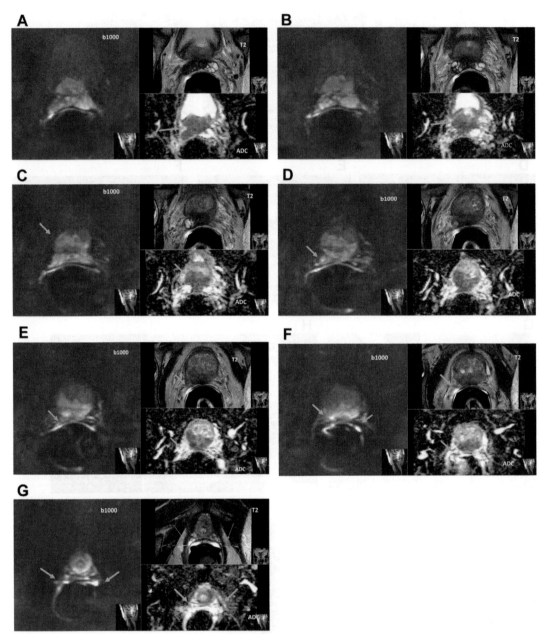

Fig. 3. (*A-D*) A 65 year old man with PSA 19 ng/ml. Gleason 9 tumor on TRUS biopsy. MRI 3T with endorectal coil. Large volume prostate cancer PIRADS 5 invading the seminal vesicles and bladder base (blue arrows) (*E-G*) MRI 3T with endorectal coil.In evaluating for posterior extraprostatic extension, the endorectal coil related artifact lowers sensitivity (blue arrows).

MRI IN SUSPECTED LOCAL TUMOR RECURRENCE

In patients who have undergone prostatectomy with or without radiation for definitive therapy and develop biochemical recurrence, MRI can be useful in identifying local tumor recurrence in a small (21%) overall percentage.[8] However, a retrospective study by Venkatesan and colleagues[27] of 195 prostatectomy patients stratified by PSA found that above a PSA of 1.5 ng/mL, 1.5 TMRI with an endorectal coil was 88% sensitive for local tumor recurrence; however, with PSA less than 0.5 ng/mL MRI was positive only 13% of the time. Local tumor recurrence on MRI manifests as focal diffusion restriction, intermediate/low T2 signal, and avid enhancing tissue in the prostatectomy bed (**Fig. 4**).

ROLE OF COMPUTED TOMOGRAPHY

CT plays a role in the initial staging of prostate cancer, evaluation for radiation treatment planning and posttreatment dosimetry, assessment for treatment-related complications, and assessment of patients with suspected biochemical recurrence for metastatic disease.

PROSTATE CANCER STAGING AND COMPUTED TOMOGRAPHY

CT is a widely available fast imaging tool that is useful in the staging of prostate cancer because of its ability to detect hepatic, pulmonary, some nodal, and most osseous metastasis. It is performed in patients with intermediate unfavorable and high-risk disease and symptomatic patients with lower-risk disease.[1]

Excluding nodal metastasis, the most common prostate cancer metastases are bone, liver, and lung.[12] Clinically evident liver metastases are identified in up to 25% of patients with prostate cancer and are associated with worsened prognosis with the lowest overall median survival of 13.5 months compared with any other metastatic site, followed by lung with 19.5 month median survival.[12] Hepatic metastases are hypo-vascular and typically appear as hypo-attenuating masses on contrast-enhanced imaging in all phases. Lung metastases characteristically appear as well-defined variably sized smooth nodules. Osseous metastases is more commonly osteoblastic than osteolytic, but is better characterized by bone scan (**Fig. 5**).

LYMPH-NODE METASTASIS: COMPUTED TOMOGRAPHY AND MRI

Unfortunately, multiple studies have shown that CT and MRI sensitivity for metastatic lymph nodes based on size criteria of 1 cm short-axis dimension is less than 40%.[5] This is because of the high incidence of nodal micrometastases in prostate cancer and overlap in size between reactive benign nodes and metastatic lymph nodes. In addition, on MRI there is a significant overlap between ADC values of benign and metastatic lymph nodes. Given these facts, surgical lymph-node dissection remains the gold standard for identifying nodal metastasis. Imaging techniques that combine anatomic and physiologic information for imaging of pelvic lymph nodes are needed for successful prostate cancer nodal staging.[24]

MRI sensitivity can be improved by using contrast agents containing lymphotrophic ultrasmall superparamagnetic iron oxide (USPIO) nanoparticles that have uptake in the normal nodal subcapsular macrophages. The iron oxide in the USPIO results in susceptibility artifact rendering the normal lymph nodes low signal on T2 and T2*imaging and high signal on T1 secondary to T1 shortening.[11] As a result, early tumor infiltration of lymph nodes can be seen before there is nodal enlargement by identifying regions of non-uptake. Several groups studied the USPIO agent Ferrumoxitran-10 for this purpose and it showed high sensitivity on MR lymphography in the range of 90% and specificity of 95%. In particular, it was sensitive in identifying lymph nodes less than 1 cm. However, a major limitation of this agent includes the need to perform pre-contrast imaging, followed by post-contrast imaging 24 to 36 hours after administration because of its slow accumulation within lymph nodes. In addition, it must be infused slowly through a filtered needle over 15 to 30 minutes, to minimize infusion-related reactions such as hypersensitivity and back pain. Adverse infusion-related reactions occurred in up to 25% of patients during phase 3 trials of this agent. This may explain why it was not further developed by the manufacturer and is currently not commercially available outside of the Netherlands. Ferumoxytol is a similar agent that is currently FDA approved as an iron replacement therapy with limited data regarding its use in metastatic lymph-node evaluation, but may play a role in the future.[5,11]

COMPUTED TOMOGRAPHY ASSESSMENT FOR COMPLICATIONS AFTER LOCAL THERAPY

CT, MRI, and ultrasound can all play a role in detecting and surveilling complications of prostate cancer therapy. However, CT and fluoroscopy are most often used in the evaluation of these patients in the United States owing to their wide availability, as well as the excellent spatial resolution of CT, and the targeted real-time imaging capability of fluoroscopy. Discussion of fluoroscopy is outside the scope of the current discussion, but it is generally used in the evaluation of leaks at the urethral anastomosis, or fistulae related to treatment.

SURGICAL COMPLICATIONS

During a radical prostatectomy, the surgeon resects the prostate and seminal vesicles and anastomoses the bladder and membranous urethra.[9] If the disease is localized, one of the neurovascular bundles can be resected leaving the other to preserve potency. Currently, robot-assisted laparoscopic prostatectomy is the standard approach. This may be preceded by lymphadenectomy in intermediate- to high-risk patients.

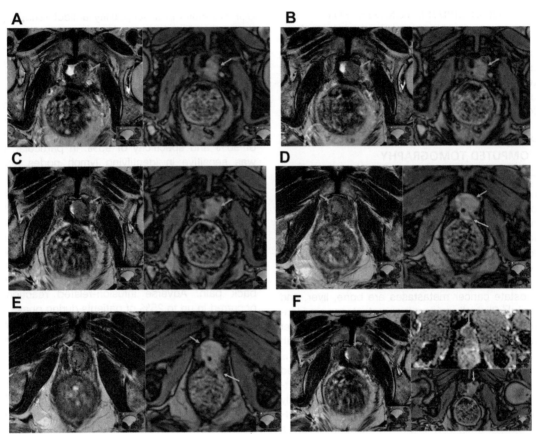

Fig. 4. (*A*) An 80–year-old patient post-prostatectomy with detectable rising PSA for 2 years. PSA 7.8 ng/mL. Findings consistent with locally recurrent prostate cancer. Lobular intermediate low T2 signal tissue, hyperintense to muscle, displaying avid early enhancement at the left bladder base and neck (*blue arrows*). (*B*) An 80–year-old patient post-prostatectomy with detectable rising PSA for 2 years. PSA 7.8 ng/mL. Findings consistent with locally recurrent prostate cancer. Lobular intermediate low T2 signal tissue, hyperintense to muscle, displaying avid early enhancement at the left bladder base and neck (blue arrows). (*C*) An 80–year-old patient post-prostatectomy with detectable rising PSA for 2 years. PSA 7.8 ng/mL. Findings consistent with locally recurrent prostate cancer. Lobular intermediate low T2 signal tissue, hyperintense to muscle, displaying avid early enhancement at the left bladder base and neck (blue arrows). (*D*) An 80–year-old patient post-prostatectomy with detectable rising PSA for 2 years now 7.8 ng/mL. Avidly enhancing intermediate T2 signal intensity tumor invading the urethra protruding into the lumen. Also note similar enhancing tissue abutting the anterior rectal wall. (*E*) An 80–year-old patient post-prostatectomy with detectable rising PSA for 2 years now 7.8 ng/mL. Avidly enhancing intermediate T2 signal intensity tumor invading the urethra protruding into the lumen. Also note similar enhancing tissue abutting the anterior rectal wall. (*F*) An 80—year-old patient post-prostatectomy with detectable rising PSA for 2 years now 7.8 ng/mL. Avidly enhancing intermediate T2 signal intensity recurrent tumor invading the bladder neck protruding into the lumen with diffusion restriction on ADC with ADC values <800.

INTRAOPERATIVE RECTAL OR URETERAL INJURY

Intraoperative rectal injury remains uncommon and reported in less than 1% of the patients. When these are not immediately recognized at the time of surgery, they typically present with fistulae to the bladder or urethra or with contained collections/abscess.[9] Imaging predominantly with contrast-enhanced CT is used in assessing for collection and/or fistula. Further confirmation with fluoroscopic imaging in some cases may be needed.

Operative ureteral injury is rare occurring in 0.1% to 0.3% of the patients undergoing robotic-assisted prostatectomy.[28] These typically occur in more technically extensive or complicated surgeries including those with bladder neck reconstruction, seminal vesicle dissection, extensive pelvic lymph-node dissection, or patients with

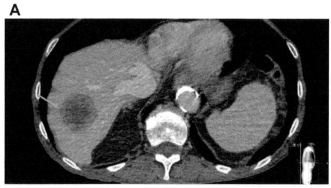

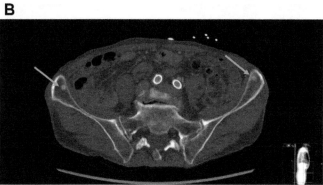

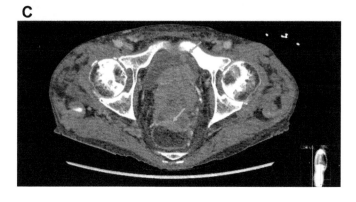

Fig. 5. (*A*) A 68-year-old man with castration resistant prostate cancer. Hypoattenuating hepatic mass compatible with prostate cancer metastasis. (*B*) Sclerotic round osseous lesions with Hounsfield unit values less than 1000 consistent with osteoblastic metastasis (*blue arrows*). (*C*). Large invasive prostatic mass. Wall thickening of the anterior rectum (green arrow) and nodule in the left anterior bladder wall (blue arrow) consistent with tumor invasion.

enlarged prostate obscuring the ureteral orifices.[28] Patients with ureteral injuries typically present in the first several postoperative days with hematuria (though this finding is absent in 25% of patients), hydroureteronephrosis, or renal insufficiency. CT with and without IV contrast with delayed excretory phase imaging or CT urogram protocol is sensitive in identifying the site of injury. Urinomas may develop at the site of injury, which manifest as simple fluid collections on non-contrast imaging, which will opacify with excreted contrast on delayed excretory phase (**Fig. 6**).

PERIOPERATIVE LYMPHOCELES

Perioperative lymphoceles occur in approximately 60% of the patients who undergo open lymph-

node dissection.[9] Most often these are asymptomatic and clinically insignificant, resolving spontaneously. However, in 2.3% of the patients, these are associated with symptoms.[9] Symptomatic lymphoceles are typically greater than 5 cm. Symptoms may result from compression of adjacent ureter or iliac veins, or superinfection. These cases will require drainage. Though these can be assessed with CT, MRI, or ultrasound, they are most often identified with CT imaging. Lymphoceles often display ovoid fluid attenuation and may have negative Hounsfield units (HU) to −18HU, related to chylous fluid. These occur in the expected location of, or immediately adjacent to, a lymph node. Infected or complicated lymphoceles will display higher HU values up to 25, and

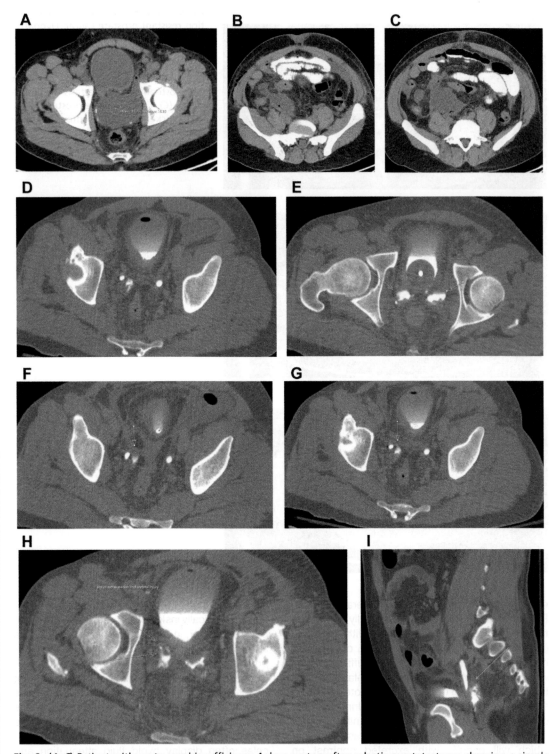

Fig. 6. (*A–C*) Patient with acute renal insufficiency 4 days postop after robotic prostatectomy, showing a simple fluid collection and few foci of gas in the recto-vesical space and tracking along the right ureter. Although gas is expected postoperatively, suspicion for urinoma is raised with low Hounsfield unit values. (*D–G*) Excretory phase mages from CT urogram 2 days after drainage catheter was placed with continued worsening renal function show contrast extravasation from the right ureter collecting in the extraperitoneal space. (*H, I*) Further images show the site of contrast extravasation and distal right ureteral injury in the surgical bed.

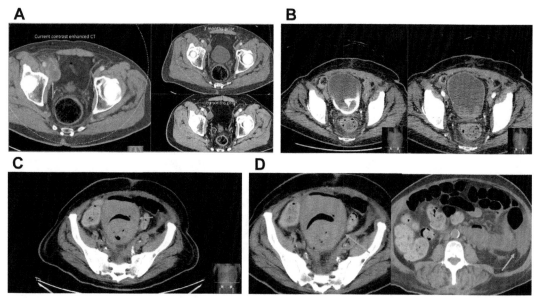

Fig. 7. (*A*) A 70-year-old man with history of prostatectomy and lymph node biopsy 9 months ago presenting with right groin pain and fever. Images on the right show a simple fluid collection along the right external iliac chain 3 months and 6 months before (*blue arrow*). On the current examination, the collection has enlarged to 5 cm with thick enhancing wall (green arrow). This was drained and noted to be a lymphocele superinfected with bacteroides fragilis. (*B*) Radiation cystitis with bladder hematoma. Non-enhancing high attenuation layering material in the dependent bladder on excretory phase on the left image and arterial phase right image. (*C*) Radiation cystitis with bladder hematoma 4 days later. High attenuation layering material in the dependent bladder consistent with hematoma and new foci of gas. More pronounced bladder wall thickening. (*D*) Radiation cystitis with bladder hematoma 4 days later. High attenuation layering material in the dependent bladder consistent with hematoma and foci of gas, left image. More pronounced bladder wall thickening (*blue arrow*). New complex peritoneal fluid related to interval bladder rupture subsequently treated with cystography.

may have increased peripheral enhancement. On ultrasound, these appear as anechoic to hypoechoic ovoid structures with occasional septae and layering debris[29] (**Fig. 7**).

RADIATION THERAPY AND RELATED COMPLICATIONS

CT, MRI, and ultrasound have continued to play a rapidly evolving role over the past 5 to 10 years in the guidance, and treatment planning, for radiation therapy. Radiation therapy for the treatment of prostate cancer is administered in several ways depending on specific patient-related factors. This can include brachytherapy with or without external beam radiation, external beam radiation therapy alone, three-dimensional (3D) conformal radiation therapy, intensity modulated radiation therapy, and a combination of androgen suppression therapy and radiation.[9]

Most complications related to prostate cancer radiation therapy are similar regardless of the method of radiation administration. These generally involve inflammation of adjacent organs including radiation urethritis, cystitis, proctitis,

rectal ulcers, fistulae between the prostate or urinary tract and rectum, and erectile dysfunction related to radiation vasculitis of the neurovascular bundle or surrounding organs. Acute proctitis and cystitis typically develop within the first 3 months and late proctitis or cystitis after 9 months.[30] There is also a risk of the late development of secondary cancer in the bladder and rectum, which increases over time from the last radiation dose. There are some additional complications, that can be specific to the route of administration. As treatment planning imaging evolves, the goal is to optimize radiation dose administration to the tumor and limit tissue damage beyond the intended treatment zone by providing the most accurate characterization of the anatomic margins of the prostate, tumor, and surrounding organs, and in the case of brachytherapy the catheters or radiation seeds.

Given the dose-related and potentially dose-limiting risk of radiation proctitis, temporary hydrogel spacers are being increasingly used. The spacer is placed through a transperineal approach into the recto-prostatic space under TRUS guidance with the intent of displacing the rectal wall posteriorly

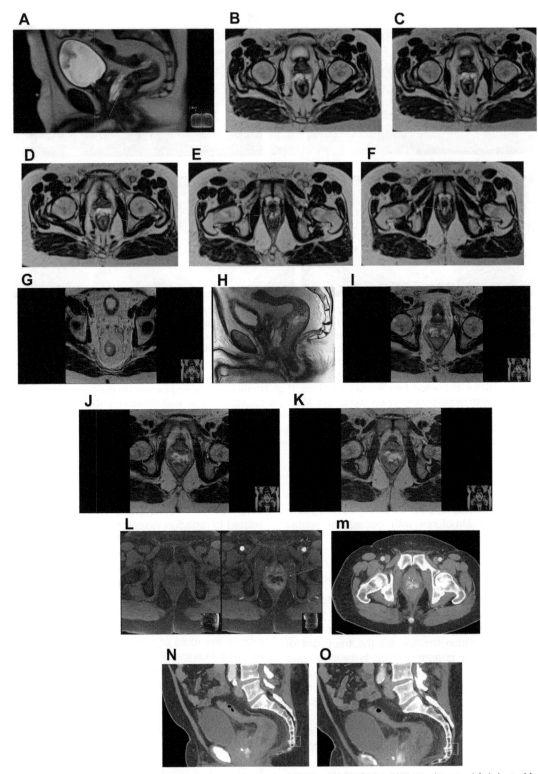

Fig. 8. (*A*) T2 hyperintense material in the recto-prostatic space on sagittal T2w MRI consistent with injected hydrogel earlier the same day. Note how the gel is seen dissecting into the anterior rectal wall to the muscularis blue arrow. (*B–F*) Hydrogel dissecting into anterior rectal wall after transperineal injection. (*G–K*) Patient returns 3 days later with severe rectal pain fever and constipation. (*G–K*) Note new presacral fluid on T2w axial and hydrogel in the rectoprostatic space. (*H*) Sag t2w image shows rectal wall edema and presacral fluid as well as the

from the prostate.[30] The spacers are typically absorbed 3 to 6 months after placement.[30] There is a risk of rectal wall infiltration by the hydrogel during placement, reported in 6% of cases during the placement of the spacer, but without an associated increase in early or late proctitis in a prospective study of 149 patients performed by Fischer-Valuck and colleagues[30,31] (Fig. 8).

With a low-dose rate brachytherapy, 50 to 125 permanent intra-prostatic radioactive seeds are placed. The seeds are cylinder-shaped shells of titanium filled with gold foil and the radioactive [125]iodine or [103]palladium and measure 4 to 4.5 mm in length $\times$ 800 μm.[32] A treatment planning CT is first performed to assess the size of the prostate and plan the number of seeds that will be needed to obtain adequate coverage of the prostate. Seeds are placed via a trans-perineal approach under TRUS guidance. With this treatment approach, the goal is to minimize radiation effect outside the prostate to adjacent organs. After the procedure, CT or MRI is performed to confirm adequate coverage of the entire prostate and intra-prostatic placement of seeds. If portions of the prostate are not covered, a second procedure may be performed. Typically, care is taken to avoid the urethra to minimize urinary symptoms although its central location makes avoidance of radiation-related symptoms nearly unavoidable and reported at a rate of 80% to 90%.[33]

During the placement of radioactive seeds in the prostate for brachytherapy, imaging with TRUS is used for guidance during the placement procedure.

Complications specific to low-dose rate brachytherapy include early edema and hemorrhage related to the seed placement procedure, loss of seeds due to passage into the urine in the first days post-procedure, and initial placement of radiation seeds outside the prostate in the surrounding tissue. When radioactive seeds are placed in an extra-prostatic location, they are most commonly found in the neurovascular bundle, levator ani, rectal wall, bladder base, seminal vesicles, penis, or obturator muscle. It has been reported that in up to 20% of the patients, radiation seeds migrate[34] into the pulmonary arterial circulation, vertebral venous plexus, and other central venous tributaries by eroding into the rich peri-prostatic venous plexus. This, however, reflects less than 1% of all implanted seeds[33,34] (Fig. 9). It is exceedingly rare for seeds migrating into the pulmonary circulation to be symptomatic, thus routine lung imaging after placement is no longer recommended by the ACR. Interestingly, there is one case report in the literature of a small cell lung carcinoma that developed surrounding a migrated prostatic radiation seed, but the causal effect was not confirmed. Case reports of myocardial infarction and radiation pneumonitis have also been published. CT continues to be the standard of care for post-implant imaging to assess dosimetry after low-dose rate brachytherapy.

High-dose rate brachytherapy is performed after treatment planning imaging to assess prostate size and contour, by inserting 10 to 20 temporary catheters under TRUS guidance into the prostate. Radiation dose, most commonly Iridium-192 is administered through these catheters periodically.

MRI-guided prostate brachytherapy has the benefit of high conspicuity of known tumor, which improves the radiation oncologist's ability to target implantation of seeds or catheters to optimize dose delivery to the site of tumor and deliver sub-volume boosting to prostate lesions that are usually inconspicuous by CT.[10] Radiation seeds can be less conspicuous on MRI when compared with CT. Some centers are performing treatment planning with an MRI-CT fusion technique, which benefits from the seed conspicuity on CT and lesion conspicuity on MRI.

ULTRASOUND

Ultrasound has been most valuable as a tool for guidance during biopsy in active surveillance patients, and during the placement of radiation seeds or catheters for brachytherapy patients. Transrectal conventional ultrasound of the prostate is neither sensitive nor specific for identifying prostate cancer. TRUS-guided biopsy of the prostate performed with 12 systematic biopsy samples (six from the right and six from the left prostate,

---

hydrogel in the rectoprostaticspace. (L) Precontrast and postcontrast 3D SPGR T1-weighted FS images show a rim enhancing hydrogel collection along anterior rectal wall and rectoprostatic space in the contrast enhanced image on the right compatible with infected collection. Patient was treated with antibiotics. (M–O) Same day CT immediately before MRI above shows the hyperattenuation of the hydrogel on CT, dissecting into rectal wall not to be confused with extravasating contrast. Rectal wall edema consistent with proctitis. Because of the high attenuation hydrogel infection could not be confirmed by CT.

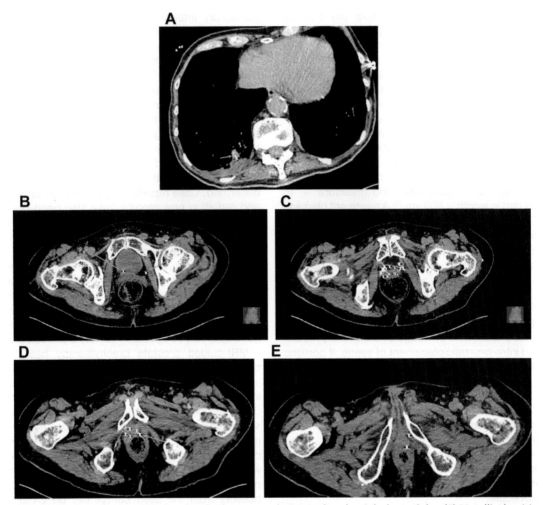

Fig. 9. (*A*) Blue arrow shows low-dose brachytherapy seed migrated to the right lower lobe. (*B*) Metallic densities consistent with low-dose rate brachytherapy seeds in bladder and left periprostatic fat. (*C*) Brachytherapy seeds in their expected location within the prostate and several migrated into the left obturator internus. (*D*) Brachytherapy seed/s in the anterior rectal wall. (*E*) Brachytherapy seeds migrated to left obturator internus and recto-prostatic space.

with two anterior biopsy samples) are standard in the setting of suspected prostate cancer. Transperineal ultrasound-guided biopsy, although less commonly performed, has been shown to be more sensitive. When mp-MRI identifies suspicious lesions (PIRADS score 3–5), additional targeted biopsy of those lesions can be performed by using software to fuse the MRI and ultrasound image and guide the urologist to the suspected lesion for additional biopsy samples. Alternatively, when such software is unavailable, the MRI and ultrasound can be cognitively fused; however, such fusion is more prone to error.

Ultrasound can play a limited role in the evaluation of immediate postoperative complications. It can be of benefit in identifying lymphoceles or identifying and following the size of postoperative collections.

Micro-ultrasound, however, in the past several years has made rapid progress, creating a potential role for the incorporation of ultrasound in the diagnostic and active surveillance paradigm of prostate cancer. In contrast to the standard ultrasound, which is performed at 6 to 12 MHz, micro-ultrasound is performed at 29 MHz with claims to increase resolution 300%[35] This superior resolution creates the ability to demarcate the zonal anatomy of the prostate. Based on early data, micro-ultrasound has been shown to have 80% sensitivity with 37% specificity for peripheral

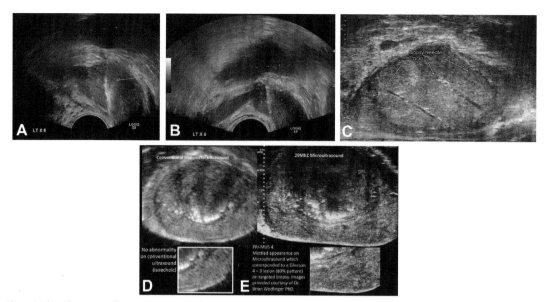

Fig. 10. (*A, B*) Images from conventional TRUS biopsy with linear echogenic needle seen within prostatic tissue (blue arrow). (*C*) Image from microultrasound performed with 29 MHz transducer shows superior resolution with needle track scars from prior biopsy. (*D*) Conventional transrectal ultrasound. No abnormality on conventional ultrasound (isoechoic). (*E*) 29-MHZ microultrasound. PRI-MUS 4. Mottled appearance on microultrasound which corresponded to a Gleason 4 + 3 lesion (80% pattern) on targeted biopsy. (*Courtesy of* B. Wodlinger, PhD, Markham, Ontario.)

zone lesions Gleason 7 and above. This technique also has the potential to lower the cost associated with an MRI first approach. The micro-ultrasound units are portable, possibly less operator dependent, and are used by the urologist in the office. The urologist can potentially identify a suspicious lesion, assign a PRIMUS score, and confidently biopsy the suspicious lesion she/he has identified. The PRIMUS (Prostate Risk Identification Using Microultrasound) protocol and risk scale is a standardized scoring scale for peripheral zone lesions based on micro-sonographic features, which has been validated and is akin to PIRADS for MRI. A recent meta-analysis of 11 studies including 1081 patients showed no significant difference between multiparametric-MRI and microultrasound in the total detection of clinically significant prostate cancer. However, the specificity of microultrasound remains low with a lower positive predictive value compared with mp-MRI. With further study and wider adoption, this modality has the potential to reduce the need for MRI and conventional TRUS/MR fusion biopsy, which is limited by cost and access. A current randomized controlled trial by Klotz and colleagues, the OPTIMUM trial, has just begun and aims to provide level 1 evidence to support the use of microultrasound in prostate biopsy by studying 1200 biopsy naïve subjects randomized to three arms: microultrasound only biopsy, microultrasound/MRI "Fusionvu" biopsy,

and MRI/US conventional fusion biopsy (**Fig. 10**). Micro-Ultrasound IMAGE GALLERY - Exact Imaging.

CLINICS CARE POINTS

- Prostate cancer management continues to evolve and currently relies on determination of a prostate cancer risk group (Low, intermediate, high) which informs shared decision making with the patient.

- MRI imaging provides the most accurate determination of T-stage in biopsy proven tumors. T-stage in conjunction with Gleason Grade group and PSA, will define the risk group assignment and help inform management approach.

- MRI provides the highest resolution in assessing for local invasion of peri-prostatic fat, seminal vesicle, bladder, and rectum. Currently MRI provides the most sensitive and accurate local staging of prostate cancer.

- The 3 most important issues to address when reporting staging prostate MRI are tumor burden (50%one side, bilateral), extracapsular extension (none, peri-prostatic fat or seminal vesicles(T3), or adjacent organs ie rectum or bladder(T4), and lymph node involvement.

- Patients who undergo surgery for prostate cancer and have ECE have poor prognosis compared to those who do not. It is advantageous in management decision making to have the most accurate assessment for ECE prior to choosing management course. MRI features most strongly correlated with ECE beyond gross tumor extension include length of tumor contact with the surface, and prostatic contour bulging or capsular surface irregularity at the site of tumor.
- MRI in an active surveillance paradigm is used to assess for development of new tumor, development of aggressive features of known tumor (including increased tumor burden, extra-prostatic extension, or lymph node metastasis).
- In Intermediate to High-risk tumors, and symptomatic patients with Low-risk disease, CT is widely used to assess for distant metastasis particularly of lung liver and lymph nodes. CT is less expensive and more widely available but less sensitive in the evaluation for osseous metastasis.
- Both CT and MRI are less than 40% sensitive in diagnosing prostate cancer lymph node metastasis by 1cm short axis size criteria alone. Surgical dissection remains the gold standard.
- Standard TRUS Ultrasound is not sensitive or specific in the diagnosis or surveillance for recurrent prostate cancer. It is mainly utilized in guidance for biopsy or guidance for treatment planning in radiation.
- Microultrasound is promising in the diagnosis and active surveillance of low risk prostate cancer with 300% resolution compared to standard TRUS and high reported sensitivity approaching that of MRI, however low specificity continues to be a challenge.
- In patients with suspected biochemical recurrence after definitive therapy, with PSA >1.5 ng/ml, MRI has been found to be 88% sensitive in evaluating for local tumor recurrence. When PSA is 0.15 MRI has been found to be only 13% sensitive in identifying a local site of recurrence.

REFERENCES

1. Barsouk A, Padala SA, Vakiti A, et al. Epidemiology, staging and management of prostate cancer. Med Sci 2020;8(3):28.
2. de Rooj M. Accuracy of magnetic resonance imaging for local staging of prostate cancer: a diagnostic meta-analysis. Eur Urol 2016;70(2):233–45.
3. Hoeks CM, Barentsz JO, Hambrock T, et al. Prostate cancer: multiparametric MR imaging for detection, localization, and staging. Radiology 2011;261(1):46–66.
4. Multiparametric MR imaging of the prostate after treatment of prostate cancer. RadioGraphics 2019. https://doi.org/10.1148/rg.2018170147.podcast.
5. Perez-Lopez R, Tunariu N, Padhani AR, et al. Imaging diagnosis and follow-up of advanced prostate cancer: clinical perspectives and state of the art. Radiology 2019;292(2):273–86.
6. Risko R, Merdan S, Womble PR, et al. Clinical predictors and recommendations for staging computed tomography scan among men with prostate cancer. Urology 2014;84(6):1329–34.
7. Stavrinides V, Giganti F, Emberton M, et al. MRI in active surveillance: a critical review. Prostate Cancer Prostatic Dis 2018;22(1):5–15.
8. Turpin A, Girard E, Baillet C, et al. Imaging for metastasis in prostate cancer: a review of the literature. Front Oncol 2020;10.
9. Yablon CM, Banner MP, Ramchandani P, et al. Complications of prostate cancer treatment: spectrum of imaging findings. RadioGraphics 2004;24(suppl_1). https://doi.org/10.1148/rg.24si045502.
10. Tharmalingam H, Alonzi R, Hoskin PJ. The role of magnetic resonance imaging in brachytherapy. Clin Oncol 2018;30(11):728–36.
11. Sankineni S, Brown AM, Fascelli M, et al. Lymph node staging in prostate cancer. Curr Urol Rep 2015;16(5). https://doi.org/10.1007/s11934-015-0505-y.
12. Ma B, Wells A, Wei L, et al. Prostate cancer liver metastasis: dormancy and resistance to therapy. Semin Cancer Biol 2021;71:2–9.
13. You C, Li X, Du Y, et al. The micro-ultrasound guided prostate biopsy in detection of prostate cancer: a systematic review and meta-analysis. J Endourology 2021. https://doi.org/10.1089/end.2021.0361.
14. Xu KM, Chen RC, Schuster DM, et al. Role of novel imaging in the management of prostate cancer. Urol Oncol Semin Original Invest 2019;37(9):611–8.
15. Leslie SW. Prostate cancer. StatPearls [Internet]. 2021. Available at: https://www.ncbi.nlm.nih.gov/books/NBK470550/. Accessed February 1, 2022.
16. Sanda MG, Cadeddu JA, Kirkby E, et al. Clinically localized prostate cancer: AUA/Astro/SUO guideline. part I: risk stratification, shared decision making, and Care Options. J Urol 2018;199(3):683–90.
17. Sanda MG, Cadeddu JA, Kirkby E, et al. Clinically localized prostate cancer: AUA/Astro/SUO guideline. part II: recommended approaches and details of specific care options. J Urol 2018;199(4):990–7.
18. Using the Cambridge prognostic groups for risk. Available at: https://www.npca.org.uk/content/

uploads/2021/02/NPCA-Short-Report-2021_Using-the-CPG-in-the-NPCA_Final-11.02.21.pdf. Accessed February 1, 2022.

19. Pierorazio PM, Walsh PC, Partin AW, et al. Prognostic gleason grade grouping: data based on the modified Gleason Scoring System. BJU Int 2013;111(5):753–60.

20. D'Amico AV. Biochemical outcome after radical prostatectomy, external beam radiation therapy, or interstitial radiation therapy for clinically localized prostate cancer. JAMA 1998;280(11):969.

21. Cvon S, Dickinson L, Pendsé D. MRI in the management of prostate cancer. Semin Ultrasound CT MRI 2020;41(4):366–72.

22. Itatani R, Namimoto T, Atsuji S, et al. Negative predictive value of multiparametric MRI for prostate cancer detection: outcome of 5-year follow-up in men with negative findings on initial MRI studies. Eur J Radiol 2014;83(10):1740–5.

23. Ahmed HU, El-Shater Bosaily A, Brown LC, et al. Diagnostic accuracy of multi-parametric MRI and trus biopsy in prostate cancer (PROMIS): a paired validating confirmatory study. Lancet 2017;389(10071):815–22.

24. Brown LC, Ahmed HU, Faria R, et al. Multiparametric MRI to improve detection of prostate cancer compared with transrectal ultrasound-guided prostate biopsy alone: the PROMIS study. Health Technol Assess 2018;22(39):1–176.

25. Rosenkrantz AB, Shanbhogue AK, Wang A, et al. Length of capsular contact for diagnosing extraprostatic extension on Prostate MRI: assessment at an optimal threshold. J Magn Reson Imaging 2015;43(4):990–7.

26. Mehralivand S, Shih JH, Harmon S, et al. A grading system for the assessment of risk of extraprostatic extension of prostate cancer at multiparametric MRI. Radiology 2019;290(3):709–19.

27. Venkatesan AM, Mudairu-Dawodu E, Duran C, et al. Detecting recurrent prostate cancer using multiparametric MRI, influence of PSA and Gleason Grade. Cancer Imaging 2021;21(1). https://doi.org/10.1186/s40644-020-00373-4.

28. Bedir F, Keske M, Demirdogen SO, et al. Diagnosis and conservative management of ureteral orifice injury during robotic prostatectomy for a large prostate with a prominent median lobe. J Endourology Case Rep 2019;5(2):39–41.

29. vanSonnenberg E, Wittich GR, Casola G, et al. Lymphoceles: imaging characteristics and percutaneous management. Radiology 1986;161(3):593–6.

30. McLaughlin MF, Folkert MR, Timmerman RD, et al. Hydrogel spacer rectal wall infiltration associated with severe rectal injury and related complications after dose intensified prostate cancer stereotactic ablative radiation therapy. Adv Radiat Oncol 2021;6(4):100713.

31. Fischer-Valuck BW, Chundury A, Gay H, et al. Hydrogel spacer distribution within the perirectal space in patients undergoing radiotherapy for prostate cancer: impact of spacer symmetry on rectal dose reduction and the clinical consequences of hydrogel infiltration into the rectal wall. Pract Radiat Oncol 2017;7(3):195–202.

32. Sachdeva S, Udechukwu NS, Elbelasi H, et al. Prostate brachytherapy seed migration to the heart seen on cardiovascular computed tomographic angiography. Radiol Case Rep 2017;12(1):31–3.

33. Nag S, Scaperoth DD, Badalament R, et al. Transperineal Palladium 103 prostate brachytherapy: analysis of morbidity and seed migration. Urology 1995;45(1):87–92.

34. Merrick G, Benson ML, Lief JH, et al. Seed fixity in the prostate/periprostatic region following brachytherapy. International journal of radiation oncology, biology, physics. 1999. Available at: https://pubmed.ncbi.nlm.nih.gov/10656395/. Accessed February 1, 2022.

35. Laurence Klotz CM. Can high resolution micro-ultrasound replace MRI in the diagnosis of prostate cancer? Eur Urol Focus 2020;6(2):419–23.

^{18}F-Labeled Radiotracers for Prostate-specific Membrane Antigen
Historical Perspective and Future Directions

Steven P. Rowe, MD, PhD[a,b,*], Ali Salavati, MD[a], Rudolf A. Werner, MD[a,c],
Kenneth J. Pienta, MD[b], Michael A. Gorin, MD[d],
Martin G. Pomper, MD, PhD[a,b], Lilja B. Solnes, MD, MBA[a]

KEYWORDS
- Radiofluorine • Radiofluorinated • Prostate-specific membrane antigen • Prostate

KEY POINTS
- Fluorine-18 is a near-ideal PET radionuclide that can provide optimized contrast resolution and spatial resolution for imaging of prostate-specific membrane antigen (PSMA).
- A number of radiofluorinated agents targeting PSMA have been developed, including the FDA-approved compound 18F-DCFPyL and other agents that may also achieve regulatory approval.
- The widespread availability of radiofluorinated agents targeted against PSMA will drive radical changes in the management of men with prostate cancer, particularly as artificial intelligence algorithms are brought to bear on large datasets.

INTRODUCTION

Much of the recent renaissance in nuclear medicine and molecular imaging[1] can be traced to the development of small-molecule inhibitors of prostate-specific membrane antigen (PSMA)-targeted agents for PET imaging of prostate cancer (PCa).[2] As those compounds entered routine clinical use in many parts of the world, ^{68}Ga-labeled agents came to dominate,[3] likely on the basis of their facile accessibility at centers that lack cyclotron-based radionuclide production.

However, it is inescapable that there are significant advantages to fluorine-18 as a radionuclide relative to gallium-68.[4,5] Those advantages include (1) well-established, centralized cyclotron production with theoretically unlimited amounts of available radiotracers; (2) a longer half-life allowing for transport to more distant centers and the development of delayed-imaging protocols; and (3) higher positron yield and lower positron energy, which lead to improved spatial and/or contrast resolution.[4,5]

As demand for PSMA imaging continues to balloon, the advantages of fluorine-18 can be leveraged to make ^{18}F-labeled agents widely accessible to patients in almost all parts of the world. A number of compounds has been synthesized and studied in preclinical and clinical settings.[6,7] In this review, we discuss the history of ^{18}F-labeled radiotracers for PSMA PET imaging,

[a] The Russell H. Morgan Department of Radiology and Radiological Science, Johns Hopkins University School of Medicine, 601 North Caroline Street, Baltimore, MD 21287, USA; [b] The James Buchanan Brady Urological Institute and Department of Urology, Johns Hopkins University School of Medicine, 601 North Caroline Street, Baltimore, MD 21287, USA; [c] Department of Nuclear Medicine, Wuerzburg University Hospital, Oberduerrbacher Street 6, 97080 Wuerzburg, Germany; [d] Milton and Carroll Petrie Department of Urology, Icahn School of Medicine at Mount Sinai, 1 Gustave L. Levy Place, Box 1272, New York, NY 10029, USA
* Corresponding author. Division of Nuclear Medicine and Molecular Imaging, The Russell H. Morgan Department of Radiology and Radiological Science, Johns Hopkins University School of Medicine, 601 North Caroline Street JHOC Room 3233, Baltimore, MD 21287.
E-mail address: srowe8@jhmi.edu

PET Clin 17 (2022) 585–593
https://doi.org/10.1016/j.cpet.2022.07.003

describe the clinical trials that led to the first US Food and Drug Administration approval of such a compound, and provide insight into the future of this class of molecules.

EARLY DEVELOPMENT OF ^{18}F-LABELED PROSTATE-SPECIFIC MEMBRANE ANTIGEN RADIOTRACERS

The first small-molecule, PSMA-targeted imaging agent was designed for PET.[8] Bearing a carbon-11, that compound, which came to be known as ^{11}C-DCMC, did not hold much translational promise but provided proof-of-principle for imaging PSMA in the periphery. Radiohalogenated radiotracers targeted at PSMA represent some of the early progenitors of the class,[9] with ^{125}I-DCIT being among the first such agents used to target PCa.[10] Although structurally similar to most subsequent PSMA PET small-molecule radiotracers, with the requisite core urea moiety bridging a glutamate to another amino acid, the 60-day half-life of iodine-125, coupled with gamma and Auger electron emissions, limited any potential clinical translation for imaging purposes. As such, effort was specifically directed at developing ^{18}F-labeled agents to obtain agents for imaging to facilitate translation.

The early and widespread adoption of ^{68}Ga-labeled agents for PSMA PET could lead one to the erroneous conclusion that ^{18}F-labeled compounds were developed later. In fact, the synthesis of the first radiofluorinated compound for PSMA PET (^{18}F-DCFBC)[11] was reported 2 years before the same group first described a ^{68}Ga-labeled radiotracer.[12] ^{18}F-DCFBC suffered from high levels of persistent blood-pool activity, but nonetheless, was an important demonstration of the ability of cyclotron-produced, urea-based small molecules for PSMA PET to identify both bone and lymph node metastases in vivo.[13,14] ^{18}F-DCFBC was found to have improved specificity for high-grade primary PCa relative to MRI[15] and also higher sensitivity for lesion detection in men with hormone-sensitive and castration-resistant metastatic PCa[14] (Fig. 1).

Another early radiofluorinated PSMA PET compound was BAY 1075553, which was particularly notable for its use of a phosphonomethyl backbone, as opposed to the more common glutamate-urea-lysine scaffold of most subsequent agents (see Fig. 1).[16] BAY 1075553 was utilized in a first-in-human study in which it was found to have lower sensitivity (42.9% vs 81.2%, respectively) but higher specificity (100.0% vs 50.0%, respectively) than the metabolic radiotracer ^{18}F-fluorocholine for lymph node staging.[17]

Of the first- and second-generation radiofluorinated PSMA PET agents, the most successful has been ^{18}F-DCFPyL.[18] ^{18}F-DCFPyL is structurally similar to ^{18}F-DCFBC but has a much more favorable biodistribution and pharmacokinetic profile, with rapid blood clearance and very high tumor uptake.[19] A secondary analysis of the first-in-human study demonstrated a markedly higher rate of lesion detection in comparison to conventional imaging.[20] The ability of ^{18}F-DCFPyL to detect subtle sites of disease underlies multiple fundamental single-center and multicenter studies.

For example, a prospective trial evaluating the role of ^{18}F-DCFPyL in preoperative staging of patients with high-risk PCa yielded encouraging results. According to the study, 28% of patients who were staged as N0 on conventional imaging had N1 disease on the ^{18}F-DCFPyL PET scan, yielding a 71% sensitivity and 89% specificity for nodal involvement compared with the histopathologic gold standard.[21] The most common reason for false positives was ureteral activity. Three patients in the study were upstaged to M1 disease with ^{18}F-DCFPyL PET. In addition to the earlier discussed findings, the study demonstrated significant agreement between the two blinded readers, suggesting high reliability of reading.[21]

A series of biochemical recurrence studies have shown that approximately 67.7% of patients with negative conventional imaging will have one or more findings consistent with a site of recurrent PCa on ^{18}F-DCFPyL PET,[22] and that the detection efficiency of the scan is correlated with PSA and PSA doubling time[23,24] (Fig. 2). Even relative to the high sensitivity of Na[18] F PET, ^{18}F-DCFPyL PET detects a similar number of bone lesions in patients with metastatic PCa.[25]

^{18}F-DCFPyL continues to be utilized in studies by a number of investigators around the world. For example, recent efforts have included studies to evaluate the patterns of change that occur in response to androgen-axis targeted agents, including abiraterone/enzalutamide[26] and bipolar androgen therapy.[27] Different groups have also studied quantitative[28] and semiquantitative[29–31] parameters with ^{18}F-DCFPyL imaging in an effort to better understand uptake variability and the potential role of ^{18}F-DCFPyL in selecting patients for different therapies and then monitoring response to those therapies.

REGISTRATION TRIALS AND REGULATORY APPROVAL OF ^{18}F-DCFPyL

The two indications for PSMA PET that have been the most extensively investigated are initial staging and biochemical recurrence.[3] As such, the two registration trials that were carried out with [18]F-

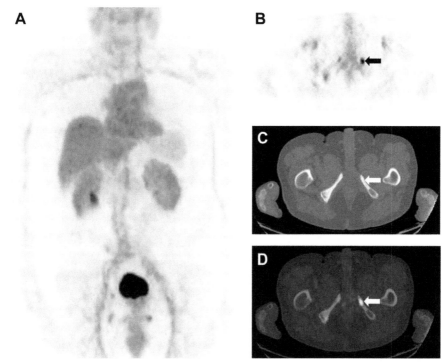

Fig. 1. A 69-year-old man with metastatic, castration-resistant PCa imaged with ¹⁸F-DCFBC. (*A*) Whole-body, maximum intensity projection (MIP) PET image. Note the significant persistent blood pool in these images obtained 2 hours post-injection. (*B*) Axial PET, (*C*) CT, and (*D*) PET/CT images demonstrate variable focal uptake in sclerotic bone metastases (*arrows*).

DCFPyL to enable a United States Food and Drug Administration (FDA) new drug application (NDA) focused on those indications. The first trial was "A prOspective phase 2/3 multi-center study of 18F-DCFPyL PET/CT imaging in patients with pRostate cancer-examination of diagnostic accuracY" or OSPREY.[32] OSPREY consisted of two cohorts, with Cohort A comprised of 252 evaluable patients with newly diagnosed, high-risk PCa who planned to undergo radical prostatectomy with an extended pelvic lymph node dissection, and Cohort B comprised of 93 evaluable patients with suspected recurrent or metastatic disease on conventional imaging who were willing to undergo biopsy.[32] The primary endpoints of the trial were sensitivity and specificity in Cohort A relative to a histopathologic evaluation of nodal involvement; the sensitivity endpoint was not met [40.3% with a 95% confidence interval (CI) of 28.1% to 52.5%] although the specificity endpoint was (97.9% with a 95% CI of 94.5% to 99.4%).[32] Cohort B generated a sensitivity of 95.8% (95% CI 87.8% to 99.0%) and a positive predictive value of 81.9% (95% CI 73.7% to 90.2%), but these were not primary endpoints of the trial.[32]

Although the specificity for lymph node involvement (one of the co-primary endpoints) and the sensitivity and positive predictive value (PPV) for

metastatic disease were all in line with expectations, the sensitivity for lymph node involvement (the second co-primary endpoint) was demonstrably lower than had previously been established in single-center trials.[21] This observation was also true in a recent ⁶⁸G-PSMA-11 multicenter trial.[33] The reasons that lymph node sensitivity in large trials remains modest and below that of single-center studies are not obvious, although they may be related to the intrinsic inhomogeneity of different scanners, scanner protocols, reconstruction algorithms, and local read paradigms.

The second registration trial was CONDOR, an evaluation of ¹⁸F-DCFPyL PET in men with biochemically recurrent PCa.[34] The primary endpoint of CONDOR was related to the correct localization rate (CLR), a variation on positive predictive value that takes into account anatomic co-localization with a truth standard.[34] Among the 208 patients in CONDOR, the median PSA was 0.8 ng/mL and 59% to 66% had at least one lesion detected on the PET scan.[34] The CLR was 84.8% to 87.0% with a lower bound of 95% CI of 77.8% to 80.4% (the prespecified lower bound of 95% CI for CLR was 20% for at least two of three central readers for the study to be considered successful). With one of two primary endpoints met in OSPREY, and the primary endpoint of CONDOR

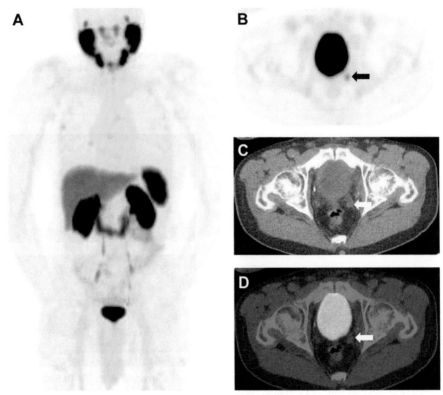

Fig. 2. A 78-year-old man with biochemical recurrence of PCa and PSA 0.4 ng/mL imaged with ^{18}F-DCFPyL. (*A*) Whole-body MIP PET image demonstrates the normal biodistribution of that radiotracer at 1 hour post-injection. (*B*) Axial PET, (*C*) CT, and (*D*) PET/CT show a site of local recurrence posterior to the bladder in the expected location of the left seminal vesicle (*arrows*).

far exceeded, an NDA was submitted for ^{18}F-DCFPyL and the agent was approved by the FDA on May 26, 2021.

EMERGING ^{18}F-LABELED PROSTATE-SPECIFIC MEMBRANE ANTIGEN RADIOTRACERS
^{18}F-PSMA-1007

An agent that has gained widespread popularity in Europe is ^{18}F-PSMA-1007. While the structure of ^{18}F-PSMA-1007 includes the glutamate-urea-lysine core moiety, its side chain/linker is composed of multiple amino acids, including one with a large hydrophobic naphthyl group, that are meant to mimic a similar structural motif on the therapeutic agent ^{177}Lu-PSMA-617.[35] That structural feature seems to contribute to unique aspects of bio-distribution and lesion specificity with ^{18}F-PSMA-1007, with minimal urinary excretion allowing for theoretic advantages in the detection of primary tumors or local recurrences[36] but high nonspecific uptake in bone lesions that can lead to erroneous diagnosis of bone-metastatic disease.[37,38]

^{18}F-PSMA-1007 PET/CT is an accurate modality for nodal staging in patients with newly diagnosed unfavorable intermediate- and high-risk PCa, with

one study demonstrating improved sensitivity and comparable specificity to whole-body MRI or CT.[39] Further, ^{18}F-PSMA-1007 has also been successfully employed in biochemically recurrent PCa, with a recent meta-analysis noting a pooled detection rate of 81.3% (95% CI 74.6% to 88.0%) that was dependent on patients' serum PSA levels at the time of the scan.[40] Given the success of ^{18}F-PSMA-1007 and wide clinical adoption in Europe, the agent has entered multicenter, phase III clinical trials in the United States and other localities (eg, NCT04742361).

[18]F-rhPSMA-7/7.3

[18]F-rhPSMA-7 is a diastereomeric mix of PSMA radiotracers that makes use of the "radiohybrid" concept that involves two different potential sites of radiolabeling (one a metal chelating site for ^{68}Ga/^{177}Lu and the other a silicon that can complex radiofluorine).[41] This allows the use of gallium-68 for diagnostic purposes, although, given the intrinsic advantages of fluorine-18, the data to date have focused on the use of radiofluorine. The compound ^{18}F-rhPSMA-7.3 is an isomerically pure version of ^{18}F-rhPSMA-7 and was used in the recent

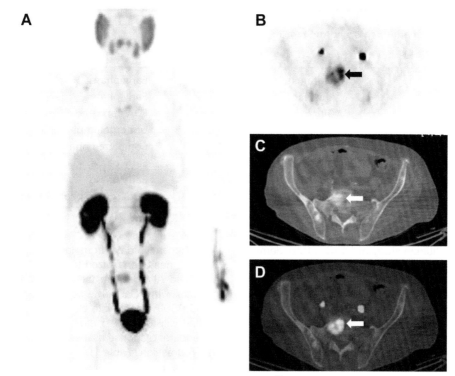

Fig. 3. A 76-year-old man with bone metastatic PCa imaged with ^{18}F-florastamin. (*A*) Whole-body MIP PET image demonstrates the normal biodistribution of that radiotracer at 1 hour post-injection, as well as abnormal uptake at multiple bony sites. There are similarities to ^{18}F-DCFPyL (see **Fig. 2**). (*B*) Axial PET, (*C*) CT, and (*D*) PET/CT show a site of bone metastasis in the sacrum with intense radiotracer uptake (*arrows*).

multicenter clinical trials SPOTLIGHT (NCT04186845) and LIGHTHOUSE (NCT04186819). The images appear to "split the difference" between ^{18}F-DCFPyL and ^{18}F-PSMA-1007, with ^{18}F-rh-PSMA-7.3 having less urinary excretion than ^{18}F-DCFPyL and fewer false-positive bone lesions than ^{18}F-PSMA-1007.

As with other radiofluorinated agents, the use of ^{18}F-rhPSMA-7 has been focused on the imaging of men with aggressive primary PCa and in the setting of biochemical recurrence. In a study of 58 patients with high-risk PCa, ^{18}F-rhPSMA-7 was found to have a sensitivity of 72.2% and a specificity of 92.5% for the detection of involved pelvic lymph nodes at the patient level,[42] similar to other agents in the single-center setting. In regards to biochemical recurrence, a study of 242 patients found that 72.7% had findings indicative of a site of recurrence, with higher detection efficiencies at higher PSA levels.[43] Given these promising results, it is likely that the SPOTLIGHT and LIGHTHOUSE trials will form the basis of an NDA with the FDA.

^{18}F-Florastamin

A promising compound with a facile synthetic approach is ^{18}F-florastamin (^{18}F-FC303). This highly hydrophilic agent has a very similar biodistribution to ^{18}F-DCFPyL and is able to detect sites of suspected PCa (**Fig. 3**).[44] To date, a phase I trial has been completed in the United States (Sheikhbahaei et al, unpublished data, 2022), and the agent is expected to be pursued in larger, prospective, multicenter trials.

^{18}F-JK-PSMA-7

^{18}F-JK-PSMA-7 is structurally very similar to ^{18}F-DCFPyL but differing in the presence of a methoxy group arising from the fluoropyridine ring.[45] This agent has been explored in multiple clinical contexts, including a study in which 70 patients being treated with androgen deprivation therapy were imaged with ^{18}F-JK-PSMA-7 PET, and 63/70 of those patients were found to have lesions with radiotracer uptake.[46] It is apparent, therefore, that ^{18}F-JK-PSMA-7 will likely continue to be explored in future studies.

^{18}F-CTT1057

^{18}F-CTT1057 occupies a unique position within this article as it is based on a phosphoramidate core instead of the glutamate-urea-lysine that is more typical of small-molecule PSMA inhibitors.[47]

Table 1
Selected information regarding the radiofluorinated radiotracers

Radiotracers	Key Chemical Moieties	Status in Prospective Clinical Trials
^{18}F-DCFBC	Glutamate-urea-lysine	Early phase
BAY 1075553	Phosphonomethyl	Early phase
^{18}F-DCFPyL	Glutamate-urea-lysine	FDA approved
^{18}F-PSMA-1007	Glutamate-urea-lysine	Undergoing phase III
[18]F-rhPSMA-7/7.3	Glutamate-urea-lysine	Completed phase III
[18]F-Florastamin	Glutamate-urea-lysine	Early phase
^{18}F-JK-PSMA-7	Glutamate-urea-lysine	Early phase
^{18}F-CTT1057	Phosphoramidate	Undergoing phase III

The first-in-human study of ^{18}F-CTT1057 demonstrated favorable dosimetry with relatively low exposure to the kidneys and salivary glands and that the agent could detect metastatic lesions with improved sensitivity in comparison to conventional imaging.[47] Currently, ^{18}F-CTT1057 is being utilized in multicenter studies involving men with newly diagnosed, high-risk PCa (NCT04838626, GuideView) and biochemical recurrence (NCT04838613, GuidePath).

FUTURE DIRECTIONS

The emergence of ^{18}F-labeled PSMA agents will allow for the eventual universal availability of PSMA-targeted imaging in all localities in which there is an existing PET infrastructure. That will mean fundamental changes in how men with PCa are managed[48] and in how imaging is incorporated into clinical trials.[49]

The improved sensitivity of PSMA PET relative to conventional imaging is driving the adoption of metastasis-directed therapy in men with limited volume metastatic disease.[50] Although true cures may be elusive in that patient population, the treatment of all visible sites of PSMA-avid disease with stereotactic ablative body radiation has been shown to improve progression-free and distant-metastasis-free survival, while also allowing men to avoid toxicities associated with systemic therapy.[48] Whether such outcomes translate into improved survival remains to be seen, but should become apparent in the future. Further, improved selection of patients for MDT through the application of artificial intelligence (AI) to patterns of disease and the delineation of whole-body tumor metrics[51] may improve outcomes relative to simple cutoffs related to the number of lesions.

Further, the entry of multiple different agents into multi-center clinical trials will lead to large datasets that will underlie rapid advancements in AI.[52] Recently, data from large trials with ^{18}F-DCFPyL has been utilized to create the first FDA-approved AI algorithm for automated staging of patients with PCa.[53] The adoption of radiofluorinated PSMA agents into clinical trials and clinical routine will further aid the adoption of AI-based methods of response assessment and monitoring for progression (**Table 1**).

SUMMARY

Despite the misconception that radiofluorinated agents for PSMA PET were developed after those labeled with gallium-68 as a means to mitigate the disadvantages of the latter radionuclide, the literature indicates that ^{18}F-labeled compounds were the first to be synthesized and their clinical development was in parallel to ^{68}Ga-labeled radiotracers. These facts underlie ^{18}F-DCFPyL (piflufolastat F18, Pylarify) becoming the first commercially available, FDA-approved PSMA PET radiotracer. As ^{18}F-labeled radiotracers drive widespread availability of PSMA PET and large clinical trials continue to be reported, these agents will transfer the care of numerous men with PCa. Innovative trial design and AI applications will help guide the future use of ^{18}F-labeled agents.

CLINICS CARE POINTS

- Radiofluorinated PSMA agents are being widely adopted for the staging and re-staging of patients with prostate cancer.
- Radiofluorinated PSMA agents have moderate sensitivity and excellent specificity for pre-operative nodal staging of men with newly diagnosed prostate cancer.

- Radiofluorinated PSMA agents have high detection efficiency for sites of disease in men with biochemical recurrence of prostate cancer.
- Future clinical applicability of radiofluorinated PSMA agents will include incorporation of artificial intelligence-driven algorithms and new imaging biomarker development.

DISCLOSURES

M.G. Pomper is coinventor on a US patent covering ^{18}F-DCFPyL and, as such, is entitled to a portion of any licensing fees and royalties generated by this technology (this arrangement has been reviewed and approved by the Johns Hopkins University in accordance with its conflict-of-interest policies). S.P. Rowe, K.J. Pienta, M.A. Gorin, and M.G. Pomper have received research funding from Progenics Pharmaceuticals, Inc., a wholly owned subsidiary of Lantheus Pharmaceuticals, Inc., the licensee of ^{18}F-DCFPyL. S.P. Rowe and M.A. Gorin are consultants for, and on the speakers bureau of, Lantheus Pharmaceuticals, Inc. M.A. Gorin is a consultant for Blue Earth Diagnostics, Inc. S.P. Rowe is a consultant for Novartis.

REFERENCES

1. Rowe SP, Pomper MG. Molecular imaging in oncology: current impact and future directions. CA Cancer J Clin 2021;72:333–52.
2. Rowe SP, Gorin MA, Pomper MG. Imaging of prostate-specific membrane antigen with small-molecule PET radiotracers: from the bench to advanced clinical applications. Annu Rev Med 2019;70:461–77.
3. Perera M, Papa N, Christidis D, et al. Sensitivity, specificity, and predictors of positive 68Ga-prostate-specific membrane antigen positron emission tomography in advanced prostate cancer: a systematic review and meta-analysis. Eur Urol 2016;70: 926–37.
4. Sanchez-Crespo A. Comparison of Gallium-68 and Fluorine-18 imaging characteristics in positron emission tomography. Appl Radiat Isot 2013;76:55–62.
5. Gorin MA, Pomper MG, Rowe SP. PSMA-targeted imaging of prostate cancer: the best is yet to come. BJU Int 2016;117:715–6.
6. Rowe SP, Gorin MA, Salas Fragomeni RA, et al. Clinical experience with 18F-labeled small molecular inhibitors of prostate-specific membrane antigen. PET Clin 2017;12:235–41.
7. Werner RA, Derlin T, Lapa C, et al. ^{18}F-labeled, PSMA-targeted radiotracers: leveraging the advantages of radiofluorination for prostate cancer molecular imaging. Theranostics 2020;10:1–16.
8. Pomper MG, Musachio JL, Zhang J, et al. ^{11}C-MCG: synthesis, uptake selectivity, and primate PET of a probe for glutamate carboxypeptidase II (NAALA-Dase). Mol Imaging 2002;1:96–101.
9. Rowe SP, Drzezga A, Neumaier B, et al. Prostate-specific membrane antigen-targeted radiohalogenated PET and therapeutic agents for prostate cancer. J Nucl Med 2016;57(Suppl 3):90S–6S.
10. Guilarte TR, McGlothan JL, Foss CA, et al. Glutamate carboxypeptidase II levels in rodent brain [125I]DCIT quantitative autoradiography. Neurosci Lett 2005;387:141–4.
11. Mease RC, Dusich CL, Foss CA, et al. N-[N-[(S)-1,3-Dicarboxypropyl]carbamoyl]-4-[18F]fluorobenzyl-L-cysteine, [18F]DCFBC: a new imaging probe for prostate cancer. Clin Cancer Res 2008;14:3036–43.
12. Banerjee SR, Pullambhatla M, Byun T, et al. ^{68}Ga-labeled inhibitors of prostate-specific membrane antigen (PSMA) for imaging prostate cancer. J Med Chem 2010;53:5333–41.
13. Cho SY, Gage KL, Mease RC, et al. Biodistribution, tumor detection, and radiation dosimetry of ^{18}F-DCFBC, a low-molecular-weight inhibitor of prostate-specific membrane antigen, in patients with metastatic prostate cancer. J Nucl Med 2012; 53:1883–91.
14. Rowe SP, Macura KJ, Ciarallo A, et al. Comparison of prostate-specific membrane antigen-based ^{18}F-DCFBC PET/CT to conventional imaging modalities for detection of hormone-naïve and castration-resistant metastatic prostate cancer. J Nucl Med 2016;57:46–53.
15. Rowe SP, Gage KL, Faraj SF, et al. ^{18}F-DCFBC PET/CT for PSMA-based detection and characterization of primary prostate cancer. J Nucl Med 2015;56: 1003–10.
16. Lesche R, Kettschau G, Gromov AV, et al. Preclinical evaluation of BAY 1075553, a novel ^{18}F-labelled inhibitor of prostate-specific membrane antigen for PET imaging of prostate cancer. Eur J Nucl Med Mol Imaging 2014;41:89–101.
17. Beheshti M, Kunit T, Haim S, et al. BAY 1075553 PET-CT for staging and restaging prostate cancer patients: comparison with [18F] fluorocholine PET-CT (phase I study). Mol Imaging Biol 2015;17: 424–33.
18. Rowe SP, Buck A, Bundschuh RA, et al. [18F] DCFPyL PET/CT for imaging of prostate cancer. Nuklearmedizin 2022;61:240–6.
19. Szabo Z, Mena E, Rowe SP, et al. Initial evaluation of [18F]DCFPyL for prostate-specific membrane antigen (PSMA)-targeted PET imaging of prostate cancer. Mol Imaging Biol 2015;17:565–74.
20. Rowe SP, Macura KJ, Mena E, et al. PSMA-based [18F]DCFPyL PET/CT is Superior to conventional

imaging for lesion detection in patients with metastatic prostate cancer. Mol Imaging Biol 2016;18:411–9.

21. Gorin MA, Rowe SP, Patel HD. Prostate specific membrane antigen targeted ^{18}F-DCFPyL positron emission tomography/computerized tomography for the preoperative staging of high risk prostate cancer: results of a prospective, phase II, single center study. J Urol 2018;199:126–32.

22. Rowe SP, Campbell SP, Mana-Ay M, et al. Prospective evaluation of PSMA-targeted ^{18}F-DCFPyL PET/CT in men with biochemical failure after radical prostatectomy for prostate cancer. J Nucl Med 2020;61:58–61.

23. Markowski MC, Sedhom R, Fu W, et al. Prostate specific antigen and prostate specific antigen doubling time predict findings on ^{18}F-DCFPyL positron emission tomography/computerized tomography in patients with biochemically recurrent prostate cancer. J Urol 2020;204:496–502.

24. Mena E, Rowe SP, Shih JH, et al. Predictors of ^{18}F-DCFPyL-PET/CT positivity in patients with biochemical recurrence of prostate cancer after local therapy. J Nucl Med 2021;63:1184–90.

25. Rowe SP, Li X, Trock BJ, et al. Prospective comparison of PET imaging with PSMA-targeted ^{18}F-DCFPyL versus Na[18]F for bone lesion detection in patients with metastatic prostate cancer. J Nucl Med 2020;61:183–8.

26. Zukotynski KA, Emmenegger U, Hotte S, et al. Prospective, single-arm trial evaluating changes in uptake patterns on prostate-specific membrane antigen-targeted ^{18}F-DCFPyL PET/CT in patients with castration-resistant prostate cancer Starting abiraterone or enzalutamide. J Nucl Med 2021;62:1430–7.

27. Markowski MC, Velho PI, Eisenberger MA, et al. Detection of early progression with ^{18}F-DCFPyL PET/CT in men with metastatic castration-resistant prostate cancer receiving bipolar androgen therapy. J Nucl Med 2021;62:1270–3.

28. Cysouw MCF, Jansen BHE, Yaqub M, et al. Letter to the Editor re: Semiquantitative parameters in PSMA-targeted PET imaging with [18F]DCFPyL: impact of tumor burden on normal organ uptake. Mol Imaging Biol 2020;22:15–7.

29. Li X, Rowe SP, Leal JP, et al. Semiquantitative parameters in PSMA-targeted PET imaging with ^{18}F-DCFPyL: variability in normal-organ uptake. J Nucl Med 2017;58:942–6.

30. Sahakyan K, Li X, Lodge MA, et al. Semiquantitative parameters in PSMA-targeted PET imaging with [18F]DCFPyL: intrapatient and interpatient variability of normal organ uptake. Mol Imaging Biol 2020;22:181–9.

31. Werner RA, Bundschuh RA, Bundschuh L, et al. Semiquantitative parameters in PSMA-targeted

PET imaging with [18F]DCFPyL: impact of tumor burden on normal organ uptake. Mol Imaging Biol 2020;22:190–7.

32. Pienta KJ, Gorin MA, Rowe SP, et al. A phase 2/3 prospective multicenter study of the diagnostic accuracy of prostate specific membrane antigen PET/CT with ^{18}F-DCFPyL in prostate cancer patients (OSPREY). J Urol 2021;206:52–61.

33. Hope TA, Eiber M, Armstrong WR, et al. Diagnostic accuracy of 68Ga-PSMA-11 PET for pelvic nodal metastasis detection prior to radical prostatectomy and pelvic lymph node dissection: a multicenter prospective phase 3 imaging trial. JAMA Oncol 2021;7:1635–42.

34. Morris MJ, Rowe SP, Gorin MA, et al. Diagnostic performance of ^{18}F-DCFPyL-PET/CT in men with biochemically recurrent prostate cancer: results from the CONDOR phase III, multicenter study. Clin Cancer Res 2021;27:3674–82.

35. Giesel FL, Cardinale J, Schäfer M, et al. ^{18}F-labelled PSMA-1007 shows similarity in structure, biodistribution and tumour uptake to the theragnostic compound PSMA-617. Eur J Nucl Med Mol Imaging 2016;43:1929–30.

36. Giesel FL, Will L, Lawal I, et al. Intraindividual comparison of ^{18}F-PSMA-1007 and ^{18}F-DCFPyL PET/CT in the prospective evaluation of patients with newly diagnosed prostate carcinoma: a pilot study. J Nucl Med 2018;59:1076–80.

37. Rauscher I, Krönke M, König M, et al. Matched-pair comparison of 68Ga-PSMA-11 PET/CT and ^{18}F-PSMA-1007 PET/CT: frequency of pitfalls and detection efficacy in biochemical recurrence after radical prostatectomy. J Nucl Med 2020;61:51–7.

38. Wondergem M, van der Zant FM, Broos WAM, et al. Matched-pair comparison of ^{18}F-DCFPyL PET/CT and ^{18}F-PSMA-1007 PET/CT in 240 prostate cancer patients: interreader agreement and lesion detection rate of suspected lesions. J Nucl Med 2021;62:1422–9.

39. Malaspina S, Anttinen M, Taimen P, et al. Prospective comparison of ^{18}F-PSMA-1007 PET/CT, whole-body MRI and CT in primary nodal staging of unfavourable intermediate- and high-risk prostate cancer. Eur J Nucl Med Mol Imaging 2021;48:2951–9.

40. Ferrari M, Treglia G. ^{18}F-PSMA-1007 PET in biochemical recurrent prostate cancer: an updated meta-analysis. Contrast Media Mol Imaging 2021;2021:3502389.

41. Wurzer A, Di Carlo D, Schmidt A, et al. Radiohybrid ligands: a novel tracer concept Exemplified by [18]F- or 68Ga-labeled rhPSMA inhibitors. J Nucl Med 2020;61:735–42.

42. Kroenke M, Wurzer A, Schwamborn K, et al. Histologically confirmed diagnostic efficacy of ^{18}F-rhPSMA-7 PET for N-staging of patients with primary

high-risk prostate cancer. J Nucl Med 2020;61: 710–5.

43. Rauscher I, Karimzadeh A, Schiller K, et al. Detection efficacy of 18F-rhPSMA-7.3 PET/CT and impact on patient management in patients with biochemical recurrence of prostate cancer after radical prostatectomy and prior to potential salvage treatment. J Nucl Med 2021;62:1719–26.

44. Lee I, Lim I, Byun BH, et al. A microdose clinical trial to evaluate [18F]Florastamin as a positron emission tomography imaging agent in patients with prostate cancer. Eur J Nucl Med Mol Imaging 2021;48: 95–102.

45. Zlatopolskiy BD, Endepols H, Krapf P, et al. Discovery of 18 F-JK-PSMA-7, a PET probe for the detection of small PSMA-positive lesions. J Nucl Med 2019;60: 817–23.

46. Dietlein F, Mueller P, Kobe C, et al. [18F]-JK-PSMA-7 PET/CT under androgen deprivation therapy in advanced prostate cancer. Mol Imaging Biol 2021; 23:277–86.

47. Behr SC, Aggarwal R, VanBrocklin HF, et al. Phase I study of CTT1057, an 18 F-labeled imaging agent with phosphoramidate core targeting prostate-specific membrane antigen in prostate cancer. J Nucl Med 2019;60:910–6.

48. Phillips R, Shi WY, Deek M, et al. Outcomes of observation vs stereotactic ablative radiation for oligometastatic prostate cancer: the ORIOLE phase 2 randomized clinical trial. JAMA Oncol 2020;6:650–9.

49. Schöder H, Hope TA, Knopp M, et al. Considerations on integrating prostate-specific membrane antigen positron emission tomography imaging into clinical prostate cancer trials by National clinical trials Network cooperative groups. J Clin Oncol 2022; 40:1500–5.

50. Murphy DG, Sweeney CJ, Tombal B. Gotta catch 'em all", or do we? Pokemet approach to metastatic prostate cancer. Eur Urol 2017;72:1–3.

51. Froelich JW, Salavati A. Artificial intelligence in PET/CT is about to make whole-body tumor burden Measurements a clinical reality. Radiology 2020;294: 453–4.

52. Rowe SP. Artificial intelligence in molecular imaging: at the crossroads of revolutions in medical diagnosis. Ann Transl Med 2021;9:817.

53. Johnsson K, Brynolfsson J, Sahlstedt H, et al. Analytical performance of aPROMISE: automated anatomic contextualization, detection, and quantification of [18F]DCFPyL (PSMA) imaging for standardized reporting. Eur J Nucl Med Mol Imaging 2022; 49:1041–51.

Ga-68 Prostate-Specific Membrane Antigen PET/CT: Imaging and Clinical Perspective in Prostate Cancer

Imaging and Clinical Perspective in Prostate Cancer

Ameya D. Puranik, DNB, FEBNM[a],*, Indraja D. Dev, MD[a]

KEYWORDS

- Prostate cancer • mpMRI • PSMA • PET • CRPC

KEY POINTS

- The exact utility of Prostate-Specific Membrane Antigen (PSMA) PET/CT in the loco-regional staging of prostate cancer remains unclear.
- Assessment of disease burden during biochemical recurrence and in castrate-resistant disease is of vital clinical significance.
- PSMA PET/CT is important for defining the local disease extent for planning salvage radiotherapy.

INTRODUCTION

Prostate cancer (PC) is the second most common cancer in men worldwide, with a wide spectrum of biologic behavior ranging from indolent low-risk disease to highly aggressive castration-resistant prostate cancer.[1] Traditionally, computed tomography (CT), MRI, and bone scintigraphy were used for the detection of primary, nodal disease, and distant bone metastases.[2] PC was never a primary focus when PET/CT first came into practice with Fluoro-deoxy-glucose (FDG) PET, as there was no significant glucose transporter receptor expression seen on PC cells. The 2010 to 2020 decade ushered in multiple tracers targeting PC cells, with prostate-specific membrane antigen (PSMA) being at the forefront as a transmembrane peptide which is expressed on the surface of normal prostatic tissue and overexpressed on 90% of PC cases.[3] Because of the fact that normal prostate cells and PC cells express the highest levels of PSMA, the overall expression profile is highly favorable and renders low molecular weight inhibitors of PSMA suitable for the diagnosis and therapy of PC. In 2011, Ga-68-PSMA-11 emerged as the first PET imaging agent for recurrent PC.[4] The commercial availability of Ge-68/Ga-68 generator systems and PSMA-targeting small-molecules, has led to vast clinical and imaging expertise. This has led to the emergence of newer clinical indications, which we discuss in this article.

GA-68 PSMA PET/CT
Diagnosis

Most men present with urinary retention or nocturnal frequency, for which the first line of approach is to perform an office digital rectal examination (DRE). Apart from this, a significant

[a] Department of Nuclear Medicine and Molecular Imaging, Tata Memorial Center, Homi Bhabha National Institute, Dr E Borges Road, Parel, Mumbai 400012, India
* Corresponding author.
E-mail address: ameya2812@gmail.com

PET Clin 17 (2022) 595–606
https://doi.org/10.1016/j.cpet.2022.07.004
1556-8598/22/© 2022 Elsevier Inc. All rights reserved.

number of patients are asymptomatic and are detected with high prostate-specific antigen (PSA) levels during screening, which warrants an additional work-up. Any clinical suspicion typically prompts a trans-rectal ultrasound (TRUS)-guided biopsy. Multiparametric MR imaging (mpMRI) is recommended for cases where the extent of primary is to be resolved pretreatment.[5] PSMA PET/CT is not commonly used in patients with low-risk or locally confined PC (cT1/T2). In cases where a patient presents with bone pain or symptoms suggestive of advanced disease, the clinician can order PSA assessment and simultaneous PSMA PET imaging even before a TRUS-guided biopsy due to the high suspicion of nodal and/or distant metastatic involvement.

In a study by Kwan and colleagues, the role of PSMA PET/CT was assessed in the diagnosis and staging of localized PC. All patients underwent radical prostatectomy (RP); hence, histopathology was the gold standard.[6] In this study of 72 patients, a sensitivity of 81.2% was seen for PSMA uptake at the primary site, with an average intraprostatic maximum standardized uptake value (SUVmax) of 9.0 g/mL. The highest sensitivity for PSMA uptake was found for patients with higher-grade disease and within older age groups.[6] Because the majority of the cohort belonged to ISUP Grades 1 to 3 and T-stage less than T3, the results of this study made a strong case for the utility of PSMA PET for the diagnosis of PC as an adjunct to mpMRI. It is rare that patients present with clinically occult disease that is not identified by TRUS-guided biopsy. However, focal uptake on PSMA PET along with morphologic disease observed by mpMRI can guide a more targeted biopsy and therefore help reach a more accurate diagnosis.

According to a meta-analysis, the sensitivity and specificity for mpMRI-based PC detection are 74% and 88%, respectively.[7] Berger and colleagues,[8] studied 50 male patients who underwent PSMA PET/CT for the purpose of staging in addition to mpMRI and compared the findings to histopathological diagnosis. Of the 50 primary lesions detected by histopathology, all of them were observed on PSMA PET/CT (100% detection), while 47 were observed on mpMRI (94% detection). PSMA had better sensitivity for index lesion localization than mpMRI (81.1% versus 64.8%), with comparable specificities (84.6% versus 82.7%). SUVmax of the primary prostatic site was positively correlated with serum PSA and ISUP grade. Thus, it is prudent to conclude that in routine clinical practice, PSMA-PET/CT can be advised for primary diagnosis and pretreatment work-up owing to its superior detection

of PC lesions with better sensitivity than mpMRI. However, mpMRI provides better soft tissue contrast and anatomic details, so PSMA PET/CT can be used in addition to mpMRI to provide improved detection and characterization of lesions.[9]

Locoregional Staging

T-staging

Primary prostatic site staging is often challenging to characterize owing to its small size and deep location. Early PCs that are not detected on DRE can be detected on mpMRI.[10] Use of endorectal coils, 3-T scanners, and adequate bowel preparation are very important considerations to optimize the visualization of primary lesions. Standard sequences used for prostate imaging include T2-weighted, diffusion and dynamic contrast-enhanced perfusion imaging. T1 and T2 are localized cancers, with T1 disease felt only on examination, and the T2 lesion is confined to the prostate. MRI helps in distinguishing less locally advanced primary disease (up to cT2) from disease with extracapsular extension (T3a) and/or seminal vesicle (T3b) involvement.[11] Moreover, in low-risk cancer patients, mpMRI is critical for local treatment planning, either in the form of RP or local radiotherapy.[12] PSMA PET has been studied in this area. However, because it is based on uptake pattern, the size of the primary and grade of the tumor become critical for its localization. Typically, in our practice, primary PSMA uptake is either focal or diffuse. While focal uptake is often indicative of tumor sites, diffuse uniform uptake poses a diagnostic challenge. This is primarily because benign prostatic tissue is also known to express PSMA and hence shows PSMA uptake (**Fig. 1**). Fendler and colleagues,[13] in a short series of 21 patients, evaluated the accuracy of PSMA PET to localize cancer in the prostate and surrounding tissues at initial diagnosis. In patients with biopsy-proven PC, it was observed that histopathologically positive (HP) segments demonstrated a significantly higher average SUVmax. Interestingly, in HP segments, SUVmax varied according to the Gleason score (GS), with a GS of 6 having a significantly lower SUVmax than that of a GS of 7 or greater disease, indicating that the PSMA expression at the primary site was directly dependent on tumor grade. There was no significant difference in SUVmax in segments with GS 7 or more. A SUVmax limit of 6.5 was derived by receiver operation characteristics analysis to distinguish HP from negative segments. With this threshold, PSMA PET showed 67% sensitivity, 92% specificity, 97%

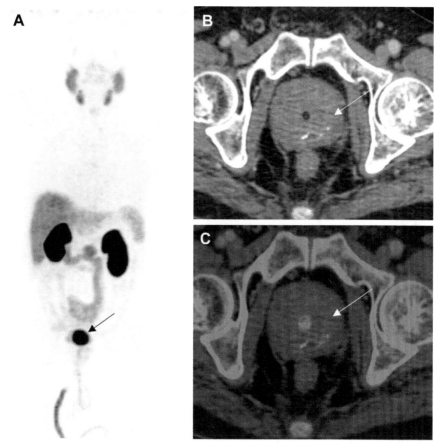

Fig. 1. A 73-year-old man presented with retention of urine since 3 weeks, DRE showed hard prostatomegaly, hence TRUS-guided biopsy was advised. PSMA PET was also done, which shows moderate prostatomegaly with diffuse PSMA uptake on axial CT (*B-arrow*) and fused PET/CT (*C-arrow*) images. PSMA uptake in the MIP image (*A-arrow*) was suggestive of physiologic urinary excretion (*arrow*). Thus, localized enlargement of prostate with diffuse low-grade uptake is suggestive of benign prostatic hyperplasia. This was confirmed on 12-core biopsy findings where all cores suggestive of benign prostate hyperplasia.

positive predictive value, 42% negative predictive value, and 72% accuracy for discrimination of HP from negative segments. PSMA PET/CT detected seminal vesicle infiltration (**Fig. 2**) with 73% sensitivity, 100% specificity, 100% positive predictive value, 77% negative predictive value, and 86% accuracy. Intense unilateral PSMA uptake is confirmatory of seminal vesicle involvement, but low-grade expression doesn't rule out involvement and can often be false-negative. PSMA PET/CT detected spread through the capsule with 50% sensitivity and 71% accuracy. However, the locoregional extent of disease can be better detected on mpMRI, as it has a definite superiority in the identification of extracapsular disease spread.

N-staging
The standard treatment algorithm for patients with non-metastatic PC is upfront surgery or local radiotherapy with or without androgen deprivation therapy (ADT). The risk of lymphatic spread is minimal for low-risk disease.[14] However, up to 33% of patients with intermediate- or high-risk disease are diagnosed with lymph node metastases (LNM). Further, LNM is proven to be a prognostic factor for biochemical recurrence (BCR)-free survival, metastasis-free survival, and overall survival (OS) in PC[15] Currently, pelvic lymph node dissection (PLND) is the gold standard for assessing lymph nodal involvement and is recommended in the scenario of high-risk PC and in cases with intermediate-risk if the estimated risk of a positive lymph node invasion exceeds 5%.[16] Unfortunately, pre-treatment conventional staging with CT and/or MRI is not particularly sensitive for the detection of LNM. Maurer and colleagues reported a sensitivity and accuracy of morphologic imaging of only 43.9% and 72.3%, respectively, in a cohort of 130 patients with prostatic carcinoma.[17] With

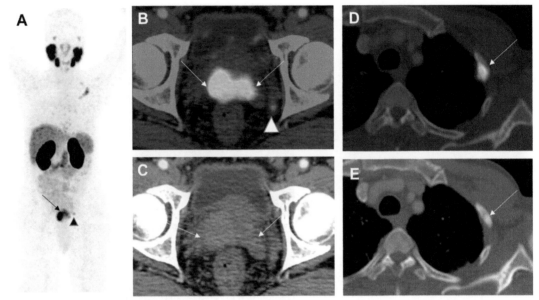

Fig. 2. A 77-year-old man presented within creased frequency of micturition and increased episodes of nocturia for 3 months. Ultrasonography showed enlarged prostate gland (Grade II prostatomegaly) with inhomogeneous echotexture. Median lobe was enlarged indenting bladder base causing mild chronic bladder outlet obstruction, with a well-defined hypoechoic lesion at the right lateral aspect of the prostate. Serum PSA levels were 129 ng/mL. mpMRI showed a nodular lesion measuring 3 × 2.5 cm in the right peripheral zone of prostate. Lesion seems hyperintense on T2W images. Marked diffusion restriction was seen. Patchy and confluent areas of hypointensity were seen in bilateral seminal vesicles suspicious for disease involvement. PSMA PET was advised, which showed intense focal uptake at the primary site on MIP image (*A*—*arrow*) and faint focal uptake adjacent to lesion (*A*—*arrowhead*). Axial PET/CT (*B*) and CT (*C*) images showed symmetric PSMA uptake in the region of bilateral seminal vesicles (*arrow*), which is seen as soft tissue thickening on corresponding CT images (*arrow*). Also seen is a discrete PSMA avid sclerotic lesion in the left third rib (*D, E*—*arrow*).

the development of modern radiotherapy protocols and cutting-edge techniques, detecting nodal involvement with greater accuracy has become critical, particularly in intermediate- and high-risk PC. As far as conventional imaging with CT or mpMRI is concerned, the cornerstone of diagnosis is based on the size of lymph nodes. Nodes with size of 8 to 10 mm are considered positive. However, metastatic pelvic nodes are frequently less than this size threshold.[18] More recently, the proPSMA randomized control trial found that ^{68}Ga-PSMA PET/CT had superior accuracy to conventional staging [CT + bone scan (BS)].[19] Moreover, the identification of positive LNM is not an isolated diagnosis but based on a combination of clinical, histologic, and imaging factors. Franklin and colleagues[20] recently published a study of 233 men who were scheduled to undergo RP with PLND. The results showed that the per-patient sensitivity of mpMRI and PSMA PET/CT to detect pelvic nodal metastases was 22.4% and 48.3%, respectively, with a specificity of 94.9% and 92.0%, with histology as the gold standard. The positive and negative predictive values for PSMA PET/CT are 66.7% and 84.3%,

respectively, compared with 59.1% and 78.7% for mpMRI. The reason for poor sensitivity was once again due to the size of metastatic nodes. In this series, histologically positive lymph nodes averaged as small as 4 mm, while those detected by PSMA PET were ≥7 mm and ≥11.7 mm by mpMRI. This emphasizes the importance of evaluation of possible LNM with mpMRI prostate imaging-reporting and data system (PI-RADS) score, PSMA PET, and other available predictive nomograms. A negative PSMA PET/CT did not reduce the risk of nodal metastases, but it did reduce the risk of LNM if the negative PSMA PET/CT was associated with a PI-RADS 4 and no seminal vesicle involvement (SVI). In a patient with a high-risk PC risk assessment score,[21] the presence of a PI-RADS 5 lesion increased the risk of a false-negative PSMA PET LNM. Another interesting finding from the study by Franklin and colleagues was based on features of the primary site, wherein a higher SUVmax, extra-prostatic extension, and SVI carried a high probability of LNM (**Fig. 3**), even if the PSMA PET was negative for nodal metastases. Overall, the predictive model from this study has identified that a

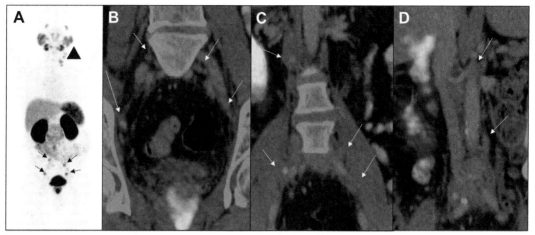

Fig. 3. A 62-year-old man presented with difficulty in voiding and a left neck swelling, which was hard on palpation. DRE: Grade IV hard nodular prostate, whereas supraclavicular node biopsy was suggestive of metastases from prostatic adenocarcinoma. On PSMA PET, MIP image shows intense uptake at primary site with PSMA avid chain of pelvic and retroperitoneal (*arrows*) and left supraclavicular nodes (*arrowhead*). This is confirmed on sagittal fused PET/CT images (*B–D—arrows*), with nodal size ranging from 7 mm to 17 mm. TRUS-guided biopsy from prostate was suggestive of conventional adenocarcinoma with Gleason score of 4 + 4. Thus, high-grade uptake with high-risk histologic features is suggestive of extensive disease, in spite of some of the nodes being less than a centimeter in size.

combination of a negative preoperative ^{68}Ga-PSMA PET/CT, ISUP biopsy grade <4 and PI-RADS <4 lesion on prostate mpMRI, or an ISUP grade 5 with PI-RADS <3 on mpMRI, is associated with a <5% risk of an LMN. Therefore, in men who are considered at risk of having a pelvic LNM, a preoperative ^{68}Ga-PSMA PET/CT and mpMRI are recommended to improve risk stratification of LNM.

M-staging

M-staging is as follows:

M1a-Nonregional lymph nodes above the common iliac artery bifurcation, as well as inguinal nodes
M1b-Bone metastases
M1c-Visceral metastases

Non-regional nodal and visceral metastases are more commonly seen in the setting of recurrent PC, and PSMA does exceedingly well at identifying such disease (**Fig. 4**). The size limitation of PSMA for non-regional nodes decreases its sensitivity. However, for visceral metastases in the liver, PSMA performs quite well. Lung metastases are evaluated purely on morphologic criteria on a breath-hold CT, as not all metastatic lung nodules are PSMA-avid. Therefore, PSMA negativity in a lung nodule does not rule out metastases, as the resolution of PSMA PET for lesion detection is 8 to 10 mm for lung nodules. The most common sites for PC skeletal metastases are the pelvic bones,

followed by vertebrae, and then other skeletal sites. Typically, a patient with intermediate-risk PC undergoes bone imaging, which includes planar BS with bone-seeking radiopharmaceutical (^{99m}Tc-MDP) or PET imaging with F18-Fluoride. PSMA PET outperforms both imaging modalities for the detection of skeletal metastases. Zacho and colleagues [22] studied 112 patients who underwent BS, mostly with supplementary SPECT/low-dose CT, and PSMA PET within less than 3 months without therapy initiation between the two investigations, and reported a sensitivity of 10% and specificity of between 93% and 96%. It is important to note that PSMA can lead to a false-positive uptake in benign bone lesions like fractures, bone islands, or other conditions. Therefore, every focus of uptake needs to be carefully examined on the CT component of PET/CT to determine its accuracy.

Treatment Response Evaluation

Assessment of response to therapy in PC patients relies on a combination of clinical parameters. The biochemical response, as reflected by a change in serum PSA levels and morphologic assessment on CT imaging using the Response Evaluation Criteria in Solid Tumors (RECIST) are commonly utilized.[23,24] Fanti and colleagues [25] led a group of researchers to create a consensus statement for PSMA PET/CT response assessment criteria in PC. The consensus statements were written with progression defined as a 30% increase of tumor

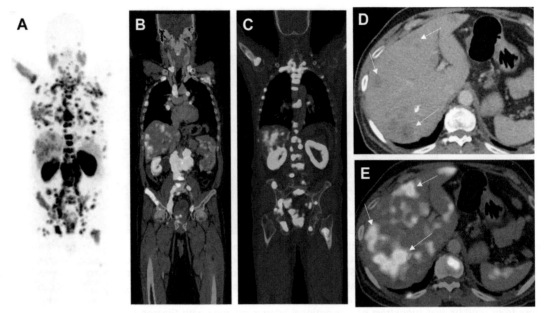

Fig. 4. A 76-year-old man presented with severe bone pain, weight loss, and difficulty in micturition. Serum PSA was 880 ng/mL and hence PSMA PET was immediately performed. MIP image (*A*) multiple foci of intense tracer uptake involving the entire body, which corresponded to diffuse nodal (*B*) and skeletal (*C*) PSMA uptake on sagittal fused PET/CT images. Multiple hypodense liver lesions (*D—arrows*) showed PMSA expression (*E—arrows*) suggestive of extensive liver metastases. Thus, PMSA PET helps in M-staging with detection of skeletal as well as visceral metastases, and even obviates the need of biopsy.

burden, which is consistent with other studies and with the modified PET response criteria in solid tumors.[26] In general, the panel defined PSMA response as follows: "complete" describes the full disappearance of any lesion with previous tracer uptake; "partial" is a reduction of uptake and tumor PET volume by >30%; "stable" is a change of uptake and tumor PET volume ≤30% without evidence of new lesions; and "progression" is the appearance of >2 new lesions or an increase of uptake or tumor PET volume ≥ 30%. One important factor is the duration between the last treatment and response scan. A potential increase in SUV measurements can be observed in a PSMA scan following initiation of ADT, due to an increase in PSMA gene expression and misinterpretation can be avoided by performing the scan no earlier than 3 months after the start of ADT (**Fig. 5**). Another challenge exists with respect to assessing response in metastatic skeletal lesions. Bone or CT scans can demonstrate persistent uptake or sclerosis, respectively, following treatment, that may interfere with the accurate assessment of the response to treatment. Absence of or reduced PSMA uptake in these bone lesions is suggestive of a treatment response (**Fig. 6**). Thus, PSMA PET accurately depicts the status of bone involvement following treatment.

Serum PSA levels have been the cornerstone of response assessment and follow-up, and parameters such as PSA50 have been associated with outcomes and used in multiple large prospective trials. In everyday clinical scenarios, however, PSA levels have demonstrated limitations (**Table 1**) with regard to their ability to accurately assess therapeutic response and do not necessarily correlate with survival. Han and colleagues[27] examined agreement between PSMA PET and PSA for response assessment in 10 studies that evaluated patients with metastatic castrate-resistant prostate cancer (CRPC) treated systemically. Though there was no conclusive evidence, PSMA PET-based volumetric parameters were good predictors of response and correlated with OS. The findings of the literature have been mixed, with 10% to 13% of patients showing discordance between PSA and PSMA response. Phenotypes emerging during progression may be manifesting clonal heterogeneity in castration resistance, which in turn would result in differential expression of PSMA and PSA-related genes, both of which are controlled, in opposing directions, by androgen receptor signaling.[28] There could also be a mixed response between different metastatic sites, which can be seen as the regression of some lesions and progression of other lesions (or the appearance of new lesions altogether). Hence, there could be a PSA response but PSMA PET-based progression of disease.[29] Neuroendocrine

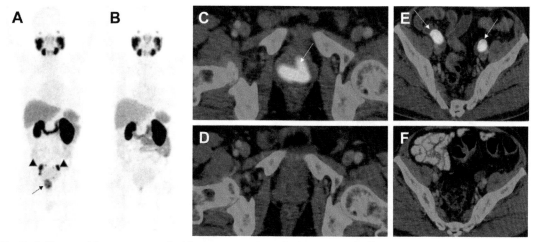

Fig. 5. A 66-year-old man presented with acute retention of urine—on and off since 6 months—USG was suggestive of moderate prostatomegaly, TRUS-guided biopsy—prostatic adenocarcinoma, Gleason score—3 + 4 = 7, baseline PSMA PET showed uptake at primary site and in pelvic, presacral and mesorectal nodes, on MIP image (primary—*arrows*, nodes—*arrowheads*). Axial PET images showed PSMA uptake in primary site (*C—arrow*) and metastatic pelvic (*E—arrows*) nodes. Patient was started on injection of leuprolide with bicalutamide. PSMA PET was done after 6 months (*B*) showed significant reduction in size and uptake at primary site (*D*), with near complete regression in size and PSMA expression in metastatic nodes (*E*) and (*F*). Thus, timing of PSMA imaging after ADT is important; also, PSMA PET helps in response assessment and thereby further adjuvant treatment can be planned.

or other dedifferentiated PCs can manifest with low or variable levels of expression of PSA and PSMA.[30]

Biochemical Recurrence

BCR is defined as two consecutive PSA values $\geq$ 0.2 ng/mL after RP or any PSA increase of 2.0 ng/mL above the nadir following radiation therapy and/or brachytherapy. However, in recent clinical trials, other definitions have been applied.[31,32] Many patients with PSA relapse who have a short PSA doubling time (PSADT) of <3 months and cancers that have a high ISUP grade, progress to metastatic cancer and cancer-specific death despite salvage treatment.

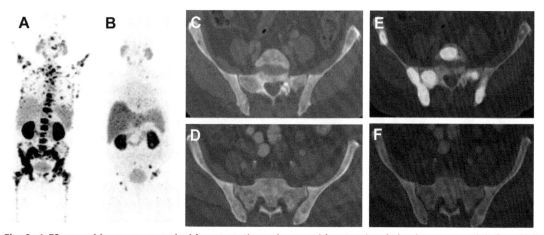

Fig. 6. A 72-year-old man presented with metastatic carcinoma with extensive skeletal metastases (*A*), for which he received upfront docetaxel, and PSMA PET at 6 months (*B*) showed significant reduction in PSMA uptake. Based on CT findings, there was persistent sclerosis on both baseline (*C*) and post-treatment (*D*) scan, however, PSMA uptake was suggestive of response to treatment (*E*—baseline, *F*—post-treatment). Thus, PSMA is an accurate indicator of response for skeletal metastases, as CT appearance of sclerosis is similar for treatment-naïve and post-treatment lesions.

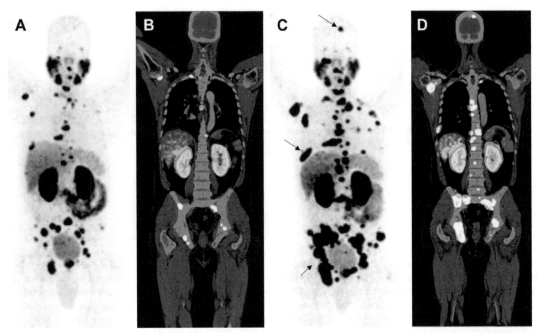

Fig. 7. A 68-year-old man, case of hormone-sensitive prostate cancer with skeletal and nodal metastases as seen on PSMA PET MIP (*A*) and sagittal fused (*B*) images. Patient received docetaxel and achieved PSA nadir, however, after 9 months, showed rising PSA levels (248 ng/mL). PSMA PET (*C*) showed increase in size and number of nodal metastases (*C—arrows*), with more than two new skeletal metastatic lesions (*C—arrows, D*) suggestive of disease progression (biochemical failure).

Compared with conventional imaging modalities, such as CT and BS, the PSMA PET scan has relatively high sensitivity, especially for patients with PSA relapse and PSA levels <2 ng/mL.[33] Today, the United States Food and Drug Administration and many guidelines recommend examination of patients with PSA relapse with ^{68}Ga-PSMA PET/CT.[34,35] PSMA PET positivity increases with PSA

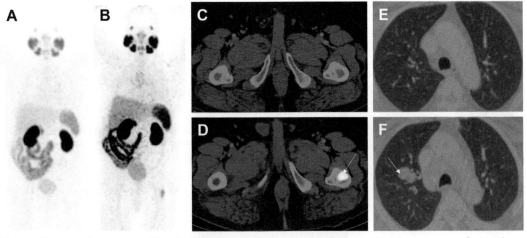

Fig. 8. A 76-year-old man, case of locally advanced prostatic cancer (T4/T3b N1 M0, Gleason score of –4 + 4), was treated with hormonal therapy, followed by radical external beam radiotherapy, achieved a serum PSA level of 0.8 ng/mL. PSMA PET done at this time (*A*) showed no PSMA expression at primary site or elsewhere in the body (*C, E*). After 11 months, presented with rising PSA levels (PSA > 29 ng/mL). PSMA PET (*B*) showed focal PSMA uptake in the proximal shaft of left femur which was a new finding (*D—arrow*), along with new lung nodules seen in lung window (*F—arrow*). This was suggestive of disease progression. Lung nodules are purely characterized on CT features, and PSMA expression may or may not be seen in metastatic lung nodules.

Table 1
Pitfalls and limitations of PSMA PET/CT

	Locations of Uptake	Misinterpreted as
False-Positive	Nonspecific reactive adenopathy	Metastases
	Asymmetric salivary glands	Lymph node metastases
	Celiac and stellate ganglion	Lymph node metastases
	Infective lung disease	Lung metastases
	Atherosclerotic plaques	Lymph nodes
	Paget's disease of bone	Skeletal metastases
	Non prostatic malignancies-lung, hepatocellular carcinoma, glioma, renal cell carcinoma	Metastatic lesions
False-Negative	Neuroendocrine carcinoma of prostate	
	Acinar cell carcinoma of prostate	
	Poorly differentiated carcinoma	

levels, with a detection rate of 57.9% for PSA levels of 0.2 to 0.5 ng/mL, 72.7% for PSA levels of 0.5 to 1.0 ng/mL, 93.1% for PSA levels of 1.0 to 2.0 ng/mL, and 96.8% for PSA levels higher than 2.0 ng/mL.[36] The current literature has shown that abdomino-pelvic lymph nodes are the most prevalent site of metastases in the BCR scenario (~50% of cases), followed by local recurrence and bone metastases (~35%).(Fig. 7) The least frequent sites are supra-diaphragmatic lymph nodes and visceral metastases (~5%). A mixed pattern of these locations may occur in about 30% of patients. The most challenging scenario is the detection of local recurrence following RP. Typically, RP relies on complete excision of the gland with the creation of a vesicourethral anastomosis between the membranous part of the urethra and the bladder. This is the most common site of postoperative local recurrence, accounting for 57%–62% of relapse cases. With PSMA PET/CT, local recurrence seems more often as a focal ill-defined hypoattenuating soft tissue mass with moderate PSMA uptake but can also simply appear as focal unilateral radiotracer uptake within fibrotic tissue. It is important to note that, in most cases, detection of post-operative local recurrence relies only on the PET component of the hybrid imaging because of the known lack of soft-tissue contrast in the pelvic region with CT or MRI. Although the PSMA component has a high lesion-to-background ratio, the prostate bed is the most difficult site to analyze because of the regional urinary radiotracer activity. There are two main explanations for this: (1) the strong urinary excretion of PSMA and (2) the relative frequency of patient urinary incontinence. Together, it leads to high radiotracer activity in the bladder/proximal urethra. To overcome this potential interference, it is recommended to (1) administer an intravenous diuretic (eg, furosemide) before image acquisition and (2) request pre-imaging voiding to reduce interference from physiologic urinary activity as much as possible, allowing neoplastic lesion uptake to be highlighted. Another recently proposed approach for better detection of local recurrence is to perform early image acquisition of the pelvic region (up to 6 minutes after tracer injection). The absence of urinary radiotracer activity at that time highlights the detection of focal uptake by tumor recurrence.[37] The existing literature on PSMA PET in BCR after radiation therapy (alone or in conjunction with ADT) is scarce. The detection rate of local recurrence in the prostate with PSMA PET after radiation therapy is 48%–63.5%.[38] Tumor recurrence seems to be associated with focal tracer uptake in the prostate or even in the seminal vesicles. It has been noted that the relapse tends to occur at the same gland location as the primary lesion before treatment. Moreover, the extent of uptake at the primary site or elsewhere also determines further treatment options. After BCR, salvage radiotherapy (SRT) is the main curative option.[39] Overall, SRT offers long-term biochemical control in about 50% of patients,[40] depending on pre-SRT PSA,[41] radiotherapy dose,[42] and risk group.[43] For high-risk patients, 5-year BCR after SRT reaches 70%.[44] Intuitively, SRT is only potentially curative if the recurrent disease is completely encompassed by the irradiated volumes. Therefore, accurate localization of recurrent disease is critical. In practice, SRT is commonly initiated in patients with serum PSA levels of less than 1 ng/mL, a threshold at which standard-of care imaging is insensitive for detecting recurrence.[45] As such, SRT target volumes are usually determined in the absence of radiographically visible disease. Callais and colleagues, in a consecutive series of

270 men, assessed the potential impact of PSMA PET for target volume delineation following early BCR (with PSA values <1 ng/mL). Fifty-two (19%) of the patients had PSMA-positive lesions not covered by the consensus clinical target volume (CTV), which would have resulted in under-treatment. Nineteen patients with pelvic LN metastasis outside the consensus CTVs (7% of all 270 patients) needed extension of CTVs to cover PSMA-expressing disease. As many as 22 of 33 patients with extrapelvic metastases (67%) were oligometastatic (<5 metastatic sites), potentially eligible for metastasis-directed stereotactic body radiation therapy. Finally, in 15% of patients, superior extension of nodal CTVs was suggested to involve para-aortic nodes.

Castrate-Resistant Prostate Cancer

According to the 2014 EAU guidelines,[46] CRPC is defined as tumor progression after a patient has undergone castration therapy, leading to plasma testosterone levels ≤50 ng/dL [1.7 nmol/L]). Biochemical progression is defined as three successive increases in PSA levels from the lowest reported PSA level, with an interval of at least 1 week in between the tests, wherein there are two increases of 50% above the nadir, with a minimum of 2 ng/mL in one of these analyses. Before a patient receiving complete androgen blockade can be classified as castration-resistant, the anti-androgen must have been previously withdrawn (at least 4 weeks for flutamide and at least 6 weeks for bicalutamide). Radiologic progression is defined as the appearance of two or more new bone lesions on the bone scintigraphy or lesions in the soft tissue according to the RECIST criteria,[47] with involvement of lymph nodes that are greater than 2 cm in size. Fendler and colleagues[48] studied 200 patients with non-metastatic CRPC, PSA > 2 ng/mL, and a high risk of metastatic disease with PSADT of 10 months and/or GS of 8, with PSMA-PET positive in 196 of 200 patients. Forty-four percent of patients had pelvic-only disease, including 24% within the local prostatic bed, and 55% had M1 disease despite negative conventional imaging. After PSMA PET, a significant proportion of patients had stage migration (Fig. 8): 24% of patients had disease confined to the prostate bed, 44% had disease limited to the pelvis, and 55% had M1 disease; M1 disease was located in extrapelvic nodes in 39%, bone in 24%, and visceral organs in 6% of patients. Thus, PSMA PET is an independent tool that can provide valuable information. It serves as an all-encompassing imaging modality, leading to optimal delineation of disease in the CRPC setting, which will best facilitate appropriate therapeutic strategies.

SUMMARY

- PSMA PET/CT has now been established as the optimal initial imaging modality for staging, treatment response, and restaging of intermediate-to-high-risk PC.
- There is a definite role for its use in the imaging of patients experiencing biochemical failure.
- PSMA PET is the investigation of choice in patients with biochemically diagnosed CRPC, promoting the optimal assessment of disease burden and facilitating proper therapeutic options.

CLINICS CARE POINTS

- Prostate-specific membrane antigen (PSMA) PET/CT should be performed in all patients with biopsy-proven prostate cancer for initial work-up to plan the treatment strategy.
- PSMA PET/CT can be used as an adjunct to regional mpMRI for assessing the extent of locoregional spread in select cases.
- False-positive uptake patterns of PSMA PET should be known while reporting these studies.
- PSMA PET/CT imaging should always be coupled with serum PSA levels in the post-treatment setting.

DISCLOSURE

The authors have nothing to disclose.

REFERENCES

1. Bray F, Ferlay J, Soerjomataram I, et al. Global cancer statistics 2018: GLOBOCAN estimates of incidence and mortality worldwide for 36 cancers in 185 countries. CA Cancer J Clin 2018;68:394–424.
2. Rowe SP, Gorin MA, Allaf ME, et al. PET imaging of prostate-specific membrane antigen in prostate cancer: current state of the art and future challenges. Prostate Cancer Prostatic Dis 2016;19:223–30.
3. Kiess AP, Banerjee SR, Mease RC, et al. Prostate-specific membrane antigen as a target for cancer imaging and therapy. Q J Nucl Med Mol Imaging 2015;59:241–68.
4. Afshar-Oromieh A, Malcher A, Eder M, et al. PET imaging with a [68Ga] gallium-labelled PSMA ligand for

the diagnosis of prostate cancer: biodistribution in humans and first evaluation of tumour lesions. Eur J Nucl Med Mol Imaging 2013;40:797–8.

5. Vapiwala N, Hofman MS, Murphy DG, et al. Strategies for evaluation of novel imaging in prostate cancer: putting the horse back before the cart. J Clin Oncol 2019;37:765–9.

6. Kwan TN, Spremo S, Teh AYM, et al. Performance of Ga-68 PSMA PET/CT for diagnosis and grading of local prostate cancer. Prostate Int 2021;9(2):107–12.

7. de Rooij M, Hamoen EH, Futterer JJ, et al. Accuracy of multiparametric MRI for prostate cancer detection: a meta-analysis. Am J Roentgenol 2014;202:343–51.

8. Berger I, Annabattula C, Lewis J, et al. ^{68}Ga-PSMA PET/CT vs. mpMRI for locoregional prostate cancer staging: correlation with final histopathology. Prostate Cancer prostatic Dis 2018;21(2):204–11.

9. Maurer T, Eiber M, Schwaiger M, et al. Current use of PSMA-PET in prostate cancer management. Nat Rev Urol 2016;13:226–35.

10. Haider MA, Brown J, Yao X, et al. Multiparametric magnetic resonance imaging in the diagnosis of clinically significant prostate cancer: an updated systematic review. Clin Oncol 2021;33(12):e599–612. Royal College of Radiologists (Great Britain).

11. Razek AAKA, El-Diasty T, Elhendy A, et al. Prostate imaging reporting and Data system (PI-RADS): what the radiologists need to know? Clin Imaging 2021;79:183–200.

12. Williams C, Daneshvar M, Pinto P, et al. Emerging role of multiparametric magnetic resonance imaging in identifying clinically relevant localized prostate cancer. Curr Opin Oncol 2021;33(3):244–51.

13. Fendler WP, Calais J, Eiber M, et al. Assessment of 68Ga-PSMA-11 PET accuracy in localizing recurrent prostate cancer: a prospective single-arm clinical trial. JAMA Oncol 2019;5(6):856–63.

14. D'Amico AV, Whittington R, Malkowicz SB, et al. Biochemical outcome after radical prostatectomy, external beam radiation therapy, or interstitial radiation therapy for clinically localized prostate cancer. JAMA 1998;280:969–74.

15. Grivas N, Wit E, Pos F, et al. Sentinel lymph node dissection to select clinically node-negative prostate cancer patients for pelvic radiation therapy: effect on biochemical recurrence and systemic progression. Int J Radiat Oncol Biol Phys 2017;97:347–54.

16. Mottet N, Bellmunt J, Bolla M, et al. EAU-ESTRO-SIOG guidelines on prostate cancer. Part 1: screening, diagnosis, and local treatment with curative intent. Eur Urol 2017;71:618–29.

17. Maurer T, Gschwend JE, Rauscher I, et al. Diagnostic efficacy of 68gallium-PSMA positron emission tomography compared to conventional imaging for lymph node staging of 130 consecutive patients with intermediate to high risk prostate cancer. J Urol 2016;195:1436–43.

18. Briganti A, Abdollah F, Nini A, et al. Performance characteristics of computed tomography in detecting lymph node metastases in contemporary patients with prostate cancer treated with extended pelvic lymph node dissection. Eur Urol 2012;61(6):1132–8.

19. Hofman MS, Lawrentschuk N, Francis RJ, et al. Prostate-specific membrane antigen PET-CT in patients with high-risk prostate cancer before curative-intent surgery or radiotherapy (proPSMA): a prospective, randomised, multicentre study. Lancet 2020;395(10231):1208–16.

20. Franklin A, Yaxley WJ, Raveenthiran S, et al. Histological comparison between predictive value of preoperative 3-T multiparametric MRI and [68] Ga-PSMA PET/CT scan for pathological outcomes at radical prostatectomy and pelvic lymph node dissection for prostate cancer. BJU Int 2021;127(1):71–9.

21. Cooperberg MR, Pasta DJ, Elkin EP, et al. The University of California, San Francisco Cancer of the Prostate Risk Assessment score: a straightforward and reliable preoperative predictor of disease recurrence after radical prostatectomy. J Urol 2005;173:1938–42.

22. Zacho HD, Ravn S, Afshar-Oromieh A, et al. Added value of ^{68}Ga-PSMA PET/CT for the detection of bone metastases in patients with newly diagnosed prostate cancer and a previous ^{99m}Tc bone scintigraphy. EJNMMI Res 2020;10(1):31.

23. Mottet N, Bellmunt J, Bolla M, et al. EAU-ESTRO-SIOG guidelines on prostate cancer. part 1: screening, diagnosis, and local treatment with curative intent. Eur Urol 2017;71(4):618–29.

24. Eisenhauer EA, Therasse P, Bogaerts J, et al. New response evaluation criteria in solid tumours: revised RECIST guideline (version 1.1). Eur J Cancer 2009;45(2):228–629.

25. Fanti S, Goffin K, Hadaschik BA, et al. Consensus statements on PSMA PET/CT response assessment criteria in prostate cancer. Eur J Nucl Med Mol Imaging 2021;48(2):469–76.

26. Pinker K, Riedl C, Weber WA. Evaluating tumor response with FDG PET: updates on PERCIST, comparison with EORTC criteria and clues to future developments. Eur J Nucl Med Mol Imaging 2017;44:55–66.

27. Han S, Woo S, Kim YI, et al. Concordance between response assessment using prostate-specific membrane antigen PET and serum prostate-specific antigen levels after systemic treatment in patients with metastatic castration resistant prostate cancer: a systematic review and meta-analysis. Diagnostics (Basel, Switzerland) 2021;11(4):663.

28. Ben Jemaa A, Bouraoui Y, Oueslati R. Insight into the heterogeneity of prostate cancer through PSA-PSMA

prostate clones:Mechanisms and consequences. Histol Histopathol 2014;29:1263–80.

29. Barbosa FG, Queiroz MA, Ferraro DA, et al. Prostate-specific membrane antigen PET: therapy response assessment in metastatic prostate cancer. Radiographics 2020;40:1412–30.

30. Parimi V, Goyal R, Poropatich K, et al. Neuroendocrine differentiation of prostate cancer: a review. Am J Clin Exp Urol 2014;2:273–85.

31. Amling CL, Bergstralh EJ, Blute ML, et al. Defining prostate specific antigen progression after radical prostatectomy: what is the most appropriate cut point? J Urol 2001;165:1146–51.

32. Cookson MS, Aus G, Burnett AL, et al. Variation in the definition of biochemical recurrence inpatients treated for localized prostate cancer: the American Urological Association Prostate Guidelines for Localized Prostate Cancer Update Panel report and recommendations for a standard in the reporting of surgical outcomes. J Urol 2007;177:540–1151.

33. Afshar-Oromieh A, Avtzi E, Giesel FL, et al. The diagnostic value of PET/CT imaging with the 68Ga-labelled PSMA ligand HBED-CC in the diagnosis of recurrent prostate cancer. Eur J Nucl Med Mol Imaging 2015;42:197–209.

34. Cornford P, van den Bergh RCN, Briers E, et al. EAU-EANM-ESTRO-ESUR-SIOG guidelines on prostate cancer. Part II-2020 update: treatment of relapsing and metastatic prostate cancer. Eur Urol 2021;79:263–82.

35. Gandaglia G, Leni R, Fossati N, et al. Prostate-specific membrane antigen imaging in clinical guidelines: European association of urology, national comprehensive cancer network, and beyond. Eur Urol Focus 2021;7(2):245–9.

36. Eiber M, Maurer T, Souvatzoglou M, et al. Evaluation of hybrid 68Ga-PSMA ligand PET/CT in 248 patients with biochemical recurrence after radical prostatectomy. J Nucl Med 2015;56:668–74.

37. Uprimny C, Kroiss AS, Decristoforo C, et al. Early dynamic imaging in 68Ga- PSMA-11 PET/CT allows discrimination of urinary bladder activity and prostate cancer lesions. Eurjnucl Med Mol Imaging 2017;44(5):765–75.

38. Hruby G, Eade T, Kneebone A, et al. Delineating biochemical failure with 68Ga-PSMA-PET following definitive external beam radiation treatment for prostate cancer. Radiother Oncol 2017;122(1):99–102.

39. Thompson IM, Valicenti RK, Albertsen P, et al. Adjuvant and salvage radiotherapy after prostatectomy: AUA/ASTRO guideline. J Urol 2013;190:441–9.

40. Stephenson AJ, Scardino PT, Kattan MW, et al. Predicting the outcome of salvage radiation therapy for recurrent prostate cancer after radical prostatectomy. J Clin Oncol 2007;25:2035–41.

41. King CR. Adjuvant versus salvage radiotherapy for high-risk prostate cancer patients. Semin Radiat Oncol 2013;23:215–21.

42. King CR. The dose-response of salvage radiotherapy following radical prostatectomy: a systematic review and meta-analysis. Radiother Oncol 2016;121:199–203.

43. Stephenson AJ, Shariat SF, Zelefsky MJ, et al. Salvage radiotherapy for recurrent prostate cancer after radical prostatectomy. JAMA 2004;291:1325–32.

44. Goenka A, Magsanoc JM, Pei X, et al. Long-term outcomes after high-dose postprostatectomy salvage radiation treatment. Int J Radiat Oncol Biol Phys 2012;84:112–8.

45. Kane CJ, Amling CL, Johnstone PAS, et al. Limited value of bone scintigraphy and computed tomography in assessing biochemical failure after radical prostatectomy. Urology 2003;61:607–11.

46. Heidenreich A, Bastian PJ, Bellmunt J, et al. EAU guidelines on prostate cancer Part II: treatment of advanced, relapsing, and castration-resistant prostate cancer. Eur Urol 2014;65:467–79.

47. Eisenhauer EA, Therasse P, Bogaerts J, et al. New response evaluation criteria in solid tumors: revised RECIST guideline(version 1.1). Eur J Cancer 2009;45:228–47.

48. Fendler WP, Weber M, Iravani A, et al. Prostate-specific membrane antigen ligand positron emission tomography in men with nonmetastatic castration-resistant prostate cancer. Clin Cancer Res : official J Am Assoc Cancer Res 2019;25(24):7448–54.

Prostate Cancer Imaging with 18F-Fluciclovine

Bital Savir-Baruch, MD, FACNM[a,b],*, David M. Schuster, MD, FACR[c]

KEYWORDS

- FACBC • Fluciclovine • Prostate cancer • PET/CT • PET/MR

KEY POINTS

- 18F-Fluciclovine PET/computed tomography is the Food and Drug Administration approved for the localization of recurrent prostate cancer.
- 18F-Fluciclovine PET can identify true positive local and extraprostatic lesions even when conventional imaging is negative.
- The positivity rate increases with higher prostate-specific antigen (PSA). However, utility has also been reported in patients with very low PSA, ie, <0.3 ng/mL.
- 18F-Fluciclovine has been reported to influence treatment planning and has positively affected outcome in a randomized controlled setting. Therefore, an 18F-Fluciclovine PET scan should be considered before salvage therapy.
- With time, prostate-specific membrane antigen (PSMA) imaging will gain dominance. Yet, 18F-fluciclovine PET will still be of value to best define local recurrence adjacent to the bladder and when PSMA PET is negative or equivocal.

INTRODUCTION

Anti-1-amino-3-[^{18}F]-fluorocyclobutane-1-carboxylic acid (^{18}F-fluciclovine) is a synthetic nonmetabolized amino acid analogue PET tracer that was approved in 2016 by the Food and Drug Administration (FDA) for PET imaging of men with suspected prostate cancer recurrence after initial treatment.[1] ^{18}F-fluciclovine enters the cells via amino acid transporters, which are upregulated in prostate cancer, and is transported most similar to glutamine, an important tumor nutrient.[2] Since its FDA approval, ^{18}F-fluciclovine PET/computed tomography (CT) has been widely used across the United States and to a lesser extent internationally (Axumin; Blue Earth Diagnostics, Ltd., Oxford, UK).

Pathophysiology and Biodistribution

As ^{18}F-fluciclovine is transported via amino acid transporters that mediate influx and efflux of amino acids, for every amino acid transported into the cell, one will be transported out and washout occurs over time, resulting in a downsloping time–activity curve.[3,4] Normal distribution of ^{18}F-fluciclovine includes intense uptake by the liver and pancreas followed by moderate uptake by the skeletal muscles, bone (red) marrow, and adrenal and salivary glands. In variants, mild-to-moderate uptake is observed in the gastrointestinal tract. In the first 4 hours after injection, only 3% of the tracer is excreted via urine. However, variable early tracer urinary excretion may occur in a minority of patients.[5]

[a] Department of Medical Imaging, Division of Nuclear Medicine, University of Arizona, Banner University Medical Center-Tucson, 1501 N. Campbell, Tucson, AZ 85724, USA; [b] Department of Radiology, Loyola University Chicago Stritch School of Medicine, 2160 S 1st Avenue, Maywood, IL 60153, USA; [c] Division of Nuclear Medicine and Molecular Imaging, Department of Radiology and Imaging Sciences, Emory University Hospital, Room E152, 1364 Clifton Road, Atlanta, GA 30322, USA
* Corresponding author. Department of Medical Imaging, Division of Nuclear Medicine University of Arizona Banner University Medical Center-Tucson 1501 N. Campbell, Tucson, AZ 85724.
E-mail address: bsavirbaruch@arizona.edu

PET Clin 17 (2022) 607–620
https://doi.org/10.1016/j.cpet.2022.07.005
1556-8598/22/© 2022 Elsevier Inc. All rights reserved.

Primary Prostate Cancer Detection and Staging

Though there is literature that supports the use of ^{18}F-fluciclovine in the characterization and staging of primary prostate cancer, these are not FDA-approved indications. Several investigators have reported higher uptake between malignant prostate cancer and normal prostate tissue, as well as a correlation between ^{18}F-fluciclovine activity and Gleason Grade.[6–9] Yet, there is also an overlap between uptake in prostate cancer and benign lesions, such as benign prostatic hypertrophy (BPH).[6,7] A recent meta-analysis of six studies reported a pooled sensitivity of 0.83 and a specificity of 0.77 for the detection of primary prostate cancer and 0.57 and 0.99 pooled sensitivity and specificity, respectively, for malignant nodal detection.[10] Exploratory work has reported the value of delayed imaging to increase the specificity of primary tumor characterization.[8] Thus, while ^{18}F-fluciclovine PET should not be used alone to guide radiation therapy to the prostate, the possibility of utilizing uptake to guide biopsy to the most aggressive lesions, possibly with ^{18}F-fluciclovine PET/MR imaging, remains an outstanding area for future investigation.

Various studies have demonstrated the utility of ^{18}F-fluciclovine PET in the initial staging of prostate cancer, especially high-risk disease, with patient-level sensitivity for nodal involvement ranging from 40% to 66.7%, and specificities of 81.0% to 100%.[11–15] The detection rate for malignant nodes correlates to the metastatic deposit size and disease burden.[11–13] Sensitivity for malignant nodal detection was 55.3% per patient and 54.8% per region in a prospective study (NCT03081884) of 57 patients with unfavorable intermediate to very-high risk prostate cancer who then had radical prostatectomy and extended pelvic lymph node dissection, with specificities of 84.8% per patient and 96.4% per region.[13] In addition, ^{18}F-fluciclovine PET demonstrated superior sensitivity compared with conventional imaging for nodal disease detection (region-based 54.8% versus 19.4%, $P < 0.01$).[13] Another trial in a similar cohort of 72 patients reported 50% sensitivity and 81% specificity per patient, with overall accuracy superior to ^{11}C-choline.[15] Although ^{18}F-fluciclovine PET has insufficient sensitivity to eliminate the need for a pelvic nodal dissection, the high specificity may be used to best select patients and to guide definitive surgery.

Recurrence

The utility of ^{18}F-fluciclovine PET in the setting of biochemical recurrence (BCR) was first reported in a pilot trial, eventually culminating in FDA approval for this indication in May 2016.[16] In the original prospective the National Institutes of Health-sponsored 115 patient single-center trial (NCT00562315) in which 93 patients met final inclusion criteria, there was an overall 82.8% detection rate with a 96.1% patient level histologic standard of truth for positive lesions.[17] In a subanalysis comparing detection rate to CT, detection rate varied with prostate-specific antigen (PSA) level; 37.5% with PSA (ng/mL) < 1, 77.8% for 1 to 2, 91.7% for >2 to 5, and 83.3% for > 5, all significantly better than CT.[18] In the prospective multicenter LOCATE trial (NCT02680041), the detection rate was similar in 213 patients with BCR: 31%, 79%, and 81% with PSA (ng/mL) of 0 to 0.5, > 0.5, > 1.0, and > 2.0, respectively, suggesting utility in a subset of patients even at very low PSA levels.[19] Interestingly, in the Emory Molecular Prostate Imaging for Radiotherapy Enhancement (EMPIRE-1) trial (NCT01666808), the disease detection rate in the ^{18}F-fluciclovine PET arm was 75.4% for PSA ≤ 1 ng/mL and 90.9% for PSA > 1 ng/mL which was significantly higher than conventional imaging.[20] In a 106 patient retrospective study, ^{18}F-fluciclovine PET outperformed bone scan in detecting skeletal metastatis.[21]

Meta-analyses for the detection of recurrent prostate cancer reported per patient pooled sensitivities of 68%–79% and pooled specificities of 68%–69%.[10,22] Yet, it is most helpful to understand the diagnostic performance of ^{18}F-fluciclovine PET with respect to region and prior therapy, rather than on a whole-body basis. In the original prospective trial, for all PSA levels, the sensitivity, specificity, positive predictive value (PPV), and accuracy of ^{18}F-fluciclovine in the detection of extraprostatic disease were 55.0%, 96.7%, 95.7%, and 72.9%, respectively.[17] The multisite study of 596 patients reported a similar PPV of 92.3% for the detection of extraprostatic disease.[23] The high PPV for extraprostatic disease characterization is important as the most critical element in deciding the appropriate treatment pathway in BCR is determining if cancer is locally recurrent or is also extraprostatic.[17]

In the original prospective trial, the sensitivity of the treated prostate or bed was 90.2%, with a specificity of 40%.[17] The lower specificity for local detection seems to be due to nonspecific radiotracer uptake in inflammation or benign hypertrophy in the intact prostate setting, similar to the lower specificity reported in primary disease. In a study of 50 prostate lesions biopsied in 21 patients with ^{18}F-fluciclovine guided transrectal ultrasound, utilizing a higher intensity cutoff of positivity and delayed imaging maximizes specificity to

84.8%.[24] In the treated intact prostate setting, biopsy confirmation of recurrence is recommended. In a recent report of a retrospective two-center study of 100 patients with BCR who underwent ^{18}F-fluciclovine PET after primary radiotherapy, the per-patient detection rate was 79%, with a PPV of 89%.[25] The same study also reported a 62% detection rate even at PSA levels below the Phoenix criteria (PSA of 2 ng/mL above nadir).

Change in Management

Demonstrating that change in management leads to a change in outcome is considered a higher level of evidence-based medicine. Yet, few imaging trials focused on outcome, utilizing rigorous standards, such as prospective randomization and predefined statistically meaningful endpoints, have been completed.

The primary outcome measure of the multicenter LOCATE trial was the fraction of patients for whom ^{18}F-fluciclovine PET altered patient planned treatment based on referring physician questionnaires completed pre- and post-imaging. Of the enrolled 213 patients, a change in management was reported in 59% (n = 126).[19] Management change was influenced by both negative (30%) and positive (70%) 18F-fluciclovine PET/CT scans. Major changes were reported in 78% (n = 98) of patients with a completed treatment regimen change. Minor changes were seen in 22% (n = 28) of patients with an altered course of treatment.

The EMPIRE-1 trial was a 165-patient randomized controlled trial designed to compare conventional imaging versus [1][8]F-fluciclovine-PET/CT to guide salvage radiotherapy in post-postprostatectomy BCR with the primary endpoint being 3-year failure free survival (NCT01666808). A 35.4% change in intention to treat management was reported for those patients who underwent [1][8]F-fluciclovine PET.[20] Most importantly, there was a significant improvement in failure-free survival at 3 years (75.5% versus 63.0; $P = .003$) and even more so at 4 years (75.5% versus 51.2%; $P = .001$) in the study arm that included 18F-fluciclovine PET/CT in addition to conventional imaging.[26] Another randomized clinical trial, EMPIRE-2 (NCT03762759), is currently accruing patients in which salvage radiotherapy will be planned either with 18F-fluciclovine or 68Ga-prostate-specific membrane antigen (PSMA) in patients with BCR post-prostatectomy with a minimum of 2-year failure-free survival as the primary endpoint.

18F-Fluciclovine PET in Clinical Practice

Ever since the FDA-approved 18F-fluciclovine, it has been widely available for patients with suspected prostate cancer recurrence without the exclusion criteria present in the prospective clinical trials, such as negative conventional imaging or androgen deprivation therapy (ADT). A retrospective 152 patient analysis of clinical practice by Savir and coworkers reported an overall positivity rate of 81% (123/152) for whole-body and 55% (83/152) for extraprostatic disease.[27] The detection rate showed a positive correlation with absolute PSA ($P < .001$) but not with PSA kinetics. Although no correlation was reported between initial Gleason group and detection rate, for every one unit of increase in initial Gleason score, the odds of extraprostatic disease increased by 49% ($P < .05$). In a 165-patient analysis by Iagaru and coworkers, an overall positivity rate of 67% was reported, with the detection rate increasing with higher PSA levels and a change in management in 62% of patients.[28]

Extraprostatic disease detection at very low PSA levels is challenging yet clinically valuable in prostate cancer management. Savir and coworkers reported in a 113 patient retrospective analysis that the positivity rate stratified by PSA levels for the localization of extraprostatic disease in BCR with PSA (ng/mL) >0–<0.2, 0.2–<0.5, and 0.5–<1 to be 30% (7/23), 44% (22/50), and 33% (13/40), respectively.[29] The majority of the reported extraprostatic disease was in pelvic lymph nodes (26%), followed by extrapelvic nodes (8%), bones (12%), and soft tissue (3.5%). Schuster and colleagues described 64 patients who had clinical 18F-fluciclovine PET/CT scans for very low PSA levels of 0.3 ng/mL.[30] The study reported an overall positivity rate of 57.8% (37 of 64). For PSA >0–<0.1, 0.1–<0.2, and 0.2–<0.3 ng/mL, positivity rates were 43.8% (7 of 16), 60.0% (15 of 25), and 65.2% (15 of 23), respectively. Similar to the Savir and coworkers' analysis, the majority of the positive lesions were within the pelvic lymph nodes (22%), followed by distant metastasis (14%).

A single-center retrospective analysis reported on the performance of 18F-fluciclovine PET/CT performed on patients undergoing ADT.[31] The positivity rate of 82% (56/68) in the ADT group was similar to the 82% (206/252) positivity rate in the non-ADT group ($P > .05$). For extraprostatic disease, a positivity rate of 60% (41/68) was reported in the ADT group versus 53% (133/252) in the non-ADT group ($P > .05$). The detection rate was positively correlated with absolute PSA ($P < .01$), yet no statistical significance was found between the ADT and non-ADT groups ($P > .05$). The authors concluded that ADT does not significantly influence the detection of prostate cancer recurrence with 18F-fluciclovine PET/CT.

Although the importance of targeting oligometastatic disease (1–5 lesions) is still under study, ^{18}F-fluciclovine PET/CT has been reported by a number of investigators to be useful in this regard.[32] A subanalysis of the LOCATE trial reported that ^{18}F-fluciclovine PET/CT was positive for oligometastatic disease in 25% (53/213) of patients, of which 79% had a change in management due to the targeting of these lesions.[33]

Preparation and Scanning

Patient preparation and scanning have been previously reported in detail.[34,35] Patients are instructed to fast (except water and medications) for 4 hours before the scan and avoid exercising for 24 hours. Nevertheless, the effect of fasting before the scan is not well established. Although the mechanism is not well understood, refraining from voiding 30 to 60 minutes before the scan may mitigate early radiotracer excretion in the urine.[5,34]

The recommended dose of ^{18}F-fluciclovine is 10 mCi (370 MBq). The radiotracer is injected intravenously in the upper extremity, arm down, while supine in the scanner, followed by a saline flush, at which time the arm may be raised. Due to the rapid kinetics of the radiotracer, it is recommended to start scanning at 4 minutes post-injection (3–5 minutes), starting from below the pelvis to the skull base. Acquisition timing (2–5 minutes/bed) and reconstruction parameters are scanner specific. The CT acquisition can be performed before or after the PET scan, with or without intravenous (IV) contrast. As IV contrast has a diuretic effect and may increase tracer washout by the urine, it is recommended to perform the CT with IV contrast after the PET acquisition.[34–36]

Interpretation

[18]F-fluciclovine interpretation has been previously described in length and is summarized in **Fig. 1**.[34,36] In general, the interpretation of ^{18}F-fluciclovine is performed with a visual comparison of the tumor to background ratio, usually the bone marrow and blood pool. For bone marrow uptake, the L3 vertebra is recommended as a reference when possible. For blood pool measurements, it is suggested to use the distal abdominal aorta. If quantitation is employed, tumor maximum standardized uptake value (SUVmax) is compared with the SUVmean of the reference background.

For the interpretation of prostate bed recurrence and lymph node involvement, focal uptake is considered suspicious if it is visually equal or above bone marrow. For less than 1 cm lesions (largest dimension/long axis), ^{18}F-fluciclovine uptake may be underestimated due to partial volume averaging.

Therefore, uptake will be considered abnormal if it is significantly above the blood pool and approaches bone marrow activity (**Fig. 2**).

For BCR after non-prostatectomy therapy, evaluation of local recurrence may be less specific due to overlapping inflammation or underlying benign prostatic hyperplasia. More focal and intense uptake (greater than marrow) is more specific, whereas moderate heterogeneous uptake (at or less than marrow) is less specific. For patients post-prostatectomy, focal uptake in the vesicourethral anastomosis and/or the lateral surgical margin/bed is suspicious for recurrence (**Fig. 3**).

For the evaluation of lymph nodes, the most common sites of recurrence will include the central pelvic lymph nodes (proximal external iliac, internal iliac/presacral, obturator, mesorectal, and common iliac lymph nodes), followed by the retroperitoneal lymph nodes. Aside from location and uptake, other factors to consider include shape (round nodes are more suspicious than curvilinear nodes), grouping (multiplicity is more suspicious than solitary), and necrosis. However, isolated metastatic lymph nodes may occur.

Liver metastatic lesions may appear relatively "colder" compared with the liver background due to high physiologic tracer uptake by the liver parenchyma. Yet, malignant uptake is commonly higher than bone marrow.[37] Therefore, it is recommended to appropriately adjust the SUV window when evaluating the liver.

Owing to physiologic radiotracer uptake by red marrow, it is recommended to applicably adjust the SUV window for the evaluation of bone. Uptake is suspicious if focal, above background marrow, and clearly seen on both the maximal intensity projection (MIP) and PET-only images.

Normal Variations and Pitfalls

As ^{18}F-fluciclovine may persist within the injected vein, a right-sided injection is preferred so as not to mistake this uptake for a left-sided Virchow's node, although co-registration with CT or MR imaging will prevent this interpretive pitfall.[34–36] Amino acid transport PET with ^{18}F-fluciclovine demonstrates less frequent and intense inflammatory activity than is present with fluorodeoxyglucose PET, yet amino acid transport also occurs in benign inflammation, especially in the postoperative setting and with chronic inflammation.[38] BPH also demonstrates nonspecific radiotracer uptake. Symmetric mild-to-moderate ^{18}F-fluciclovine activity in nodes not commonly involved by prostate metastasis, such as inguinal, distal external iliac, and axillary stations, may occur. Periurethral single or dual linear mild to moderate activity is

¹⁸F-Fluciclovine Interpretation criteria
• Focal uptake is considered suspicious if visually equal to or above bone marrow.
• For lesions < 1cm (largest dimension/long axis), focal uptake will be considered suspicious if visually significantly above blood pool uptake and approaching bone marrow uptake.
• For quantitation, lesion SUV max should be compared with SUV mean of the bone marrow and blood pool.
• If possible, bone marrow SUV mean values should be measured from the normal L3 vertebra (if L3 abnormal, use adjacent normal vertebrae).
• Blood pool SUV mean should be measured from the distal abdominal aorta.

Prostate/bed			
Non-Prostatectomy		Prostatectomy	
Due to post-radiation inflammatory changes or overlapping benign prostate hypertension, uptake within the prostate may not be specific		Common sites of local recurrence include the urethral anastomosis and lateral surgical margins/seminal vesicle bed. 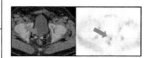 	
Focal asymmetric uptake is suspicious 	Diffuse homogeneous activity not greater than marrow usually benign 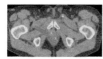		
Focal asymmetric uptake visually greater than bone marrow is suspicious and more specific than diffuse uptake. 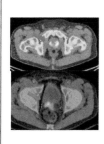	Focal uptake in lesions <1 cm abnormal if uptake is approaching marrow and significantly greater than blood pool. 	Focal uptake in a common site for recurrent disease visually equal to or greater than bone marrow is suspicious for cancer 	Focal uptake in lesions <1 cm suspicious if approaches marrow and significantly greater than blood pool 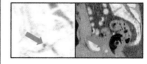

Fig. 1. ¹⁸F-Fluciclovine interpretation criteria.

commonly seen. Sagittal images are especially useful to identify recurrence at the vesicourethral anastomosis differentiated from physiologic activity.

In skeletal lesions, uptake has been described with more intensity in silent, lytic, or mixed lesions. Although sclerotic lesions also display radiotracer uptake, some indolent dense sclerotic lesions may have none or minimal activity. Mild-to-moderate solitary focal activity in the pelvis or proximal femurs may be due to activated red marrow and should not be presumed to represent metastatic disease unless confirmed by characteristic appearance on CT or ancillary bone-specific imaging, such as MR imaging, NaF PET/CT, or bone scan, preferably with single-photon emission CT.[34]

Finally, since ¹⁸F-fluciclovine reflects amino acid transport, which is not specific to prostate cancer, other benign and malignant neoplasia may have ¹⁸F-fluciclovine uptake, for example, breast, lung, glioma, lymphoma, multiple myeloma, gastrointestinal stromal tumor, meningioma, Warthin's tumor, and osteoid osteoma, among others.[38-42]

¹⁸F-Fluciclovine PET and MR Imaging

Turkbey originally described the potential additive value of separately obtained MR imaging and ¹⁸F-

Lymph nodes	
Atypical locations for lymph nodes involvement include the distal external iliac, inguinal, mediastinal, axillary, and cervical lymph nodes	Typical sites of lymph nodes involvement including the proximal external iliac, internal iliac/presacral, common iliac, aortocaval, para-aortic, and retroperitoneal lymph nodes
• Uptake within lymph nodes considered suspicious if visually equal to or greater than bone marrow 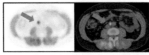 	
• Uptake is considered suspicious for lymph node < 1 cm (long axis) if it approaches marrow and is significantly greater than blood pool. 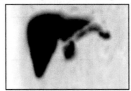	
• Multiple small < 1 cm typical lymph nodes with uptake greater than blood pool but less than marrow in typical locations for recurrence are more suspicious for malignancy than a solitary node with this level of uptake. 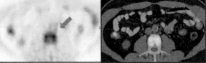	
Liver	
• Physiological tracer uptake by the liver parenchyma is high. 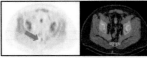	
• Metastatic lesions may appear as "cold" lesions proportionally to the liver but higher than the marrow. 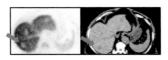	
Bone	

Fig. 1. (*Continued*)

fluciclovine PET/CT, which increased the PPV from 50% for ^{18}F-fluciclovine PET and 76% for MR imaging to 82% for the blended data.[6] The FLUCIPRO Trial Group reported that in 26 men with primary prostate cancer who underwent ^{18}F-fluciclovine PET/CT followed by PET/MR imaging, there was no statistically significant difference in prostate lesion detection between the PET techniques and mpMR imaging alone, yet PET seemed to have higher sensitivity while mpMR had the highest specificity.[9] Elschot stated that combining ^{18}F-fluciclovine PET and MR imaging parameters yielded a significantly higher area under the curve

in distinguishing tumor from benign tissue and high-grade tumor from other tissue than either PET or MR imaging alone, and that the addition of delayed PET imaging may also provide added value.[8,43] Thus, for detection of cancer in the prostate, adjunct use of MR imaging and ^{18}F-fluciclovine PET may have an additive value.

For staging high-risk primary prostate cancer, a 28-patient study evaluated the detection of malignant lymph nodes using hybrid PET/MR imaging and demonstrated similar per-patient sensitivity of 40% for ^{18}F-fluciclovine PET and MR imaging alone. Yet, PET had higher specificity (100%

- Focal uptake above the bone marrow in silent, lytic, or mixed lesions clearly visualized on PET and MIP images is considered suspicious for cancer.

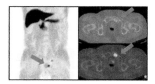

- The absence of uptake in dense suspicious sclerotic lesions does not exclude metastatic disease. Bone specific imaging is recommended.

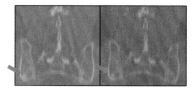

Fig. 1. (Continued)

versus 87.5) and PPV (100% versus 66.7%) than MR imaging.[12] In a recent study of 14 patients with high-risk prostate cancer staged with hybrid 18F-fluciclovine PET/MR imaging, all biopsy-proven prostate lesions were detected with PET/MR imaging. While MR imaging detected only three patients with nodal spread, seven patients were detected with PET/MR imaging.[44] Other studies comparing detection rates in recurrent prostate cancer with 18F-fluciclovine PET/MR imaging either combined or separately found no statistically significant differences between 18F-fluciclovine PET/MR imaging and MR imaging alone. However, the authors report that both modalities may have complementary utility for a more definitive diagnosis.[45,46]

Although combined 18F-fluciclovine PET/MR imaging has shown promise in the evaluation of prostate cancer, more studies are necessary. Owing to the fast kinetics of 18F-fluciclovine, it is critical to

have a PET/MR imaging protocol that leverages the recommended acquisition protocol of this radiotracer, including starting PET acquisition within 3 to 5 minutes of injection and not using a prolonged acquisition time per bed position. An example of a successful protocol in use at Emory University is presented in **Fig. 4**, along with examples of studies in **Fig. 5**.

18F-Fluciclovine in the Prostate-Specific Membrane Antigen World

Now that multiple PSMA radiotracers have been FDA approved and are in various stages of commercialization, including 18F-DCFPyL (piflufolastat F-18 or PYLARIFY; Lantheus, N. Billerica, MA), and 68Ga-PSMA-11 (UCLA/UCSF and Illuccix; Telix Pharmaceuticals Ltd., Melbourne, Australia), a relevant question to ask is what the potential uses of 18F-fluciclovine PET are in the "world of PSMA."

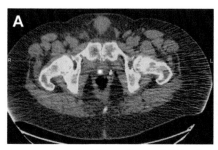
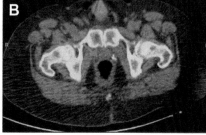

Fig. 2. A patient presented with an elevated PSA of 1.47 ng/mL after prior prostatectomy and salvage external beam radiation therapy. (A) An 18F-fluciclovine PET/CT scan demonstrated intense focus of uptake within the prostate bed suspicious for local recurrence. (B) 18F-FDG PET/CT scan was falsely negative for the localization of local recurrence.

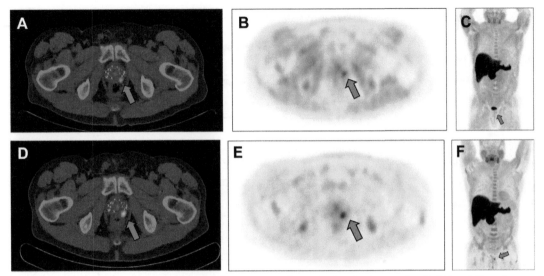

Fig. 3. A 63-year-old man with elevated PSA of 4.45 ng/mL after prior brachytherapy (nadir 0.7 mg/dL) underwent ^{18}F-fluciclovine PET/CT. PET/CT (A), PET (B), and MIP (C) images demonstrate suspicious uptake within the left posterior prostate adjoining the left seminal vesical (arrows). The lesion was confirmed positive for local recurrence by biopsy. The patient was placed on surveillance. Two years after, PSA increased to 9.8 ng/mL. The patient underwent a second ^{18}F-fluciclovine scan (D, E), which demonstrated persistent abnormal uptake left posterior prostate adjoining the left seminal vesical with interval increased intensity. The patient subsequently underwent high dose radiation salvage brachytherapy (F). Following PSA decreased to 1.9 ng/mL (below nadir + 2).

Each radiotracer probes different aspects of the biology of prostate cancer: ^{18}F-fluciclovine that of tumor metabolism as reflected in amino acid transport, and PSMA as reflected in receptor upregulation/expression. It is worth noting that while ^{18}F-fluciclovine is FDA approved for BCR only, the PSMA radiotracers are FDA approved for BCR and potential metastatic disease in higher-risk primary prostate cancer.[1,47–49] Moreover, the National Comprehensive Cancer Network guidelines now include both ^{68}Ga-PSMA and ^{18}F-DCFPyL in the staging of unfavorable intermediate-risk or higher-risk primary prostate cancer and BCR with the notation that the PSMA PET radiotracers may be used instead of conventional imaging. ^{18}F-fluciclovine does not have this endorsement and is only included in the algorithm for BCR.[50]

AXUMIN PROSTATE PET/MR PROTOCOL

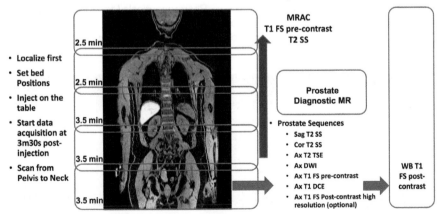

Fig. 4. PET-MR imaging ^{18}F-fluciclovine acquisition workflow for prostate cancer in use at Emory University with the Signa PET-MR imaging (GE HealthCare, Chicago, Illinois). DCE, dynamic contrast enhanced; DWI, diffusion weighted imaging; FS, fat suppressed; MRAC, MR attenuation correction; SS, single shot; TSE, turbo spin echo. (*Courtesy of* S Tajmir, MD, Atlanta, Georgia.)

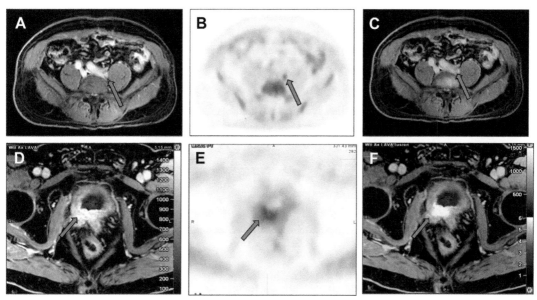

Fig. 5. Axial T1 post-contrast MR imaging (*A*), ¹⁸F-fluciclovine PET (*B*), and fused PET-MR imaging (*C*) demonstrating abnormal uptake in a 4 mm left junctional lymph node (arrows) in a patient with BCR, too small to be considered suspicious on MR imaging alone. In a different patient with BCR after radiation and cryoablation recurrence is seen along the peripheral margin of the ablation zone with bladder base invasion (arrows) on axial T1 post-contrast MR imaging (*D*), 18F-fluciclovine PET (*E*), and fused PET-MR imaging (*F*). Courtesy of S Tajmir, MD, Atlanta, Georgia.

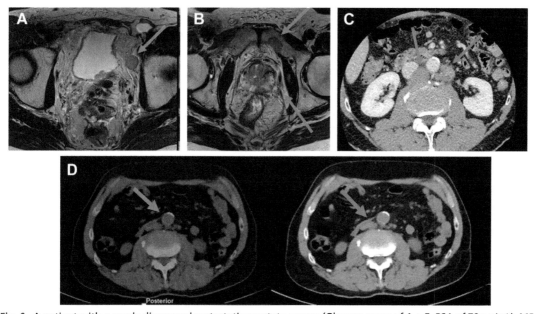

Fig. 6. A patient with a newly diagnosed metastatic prostate cancer (Gleason score of 4 + 5, PSA of 79 ng/mL). MR imaging (*A, B*) of the prostate on initial staging images demonstrated a left pubic osseous metastatic lesion with metastatic left external iliac lymph nodes (arrows). A CT scan of the abdomen (*C*) demonstrated retroperitoneal metastatic lymph nodes. The patient was started on systemic hormonal therapy with a 0.26 ng/mL nadir PSA. While on hormonal therapy, PSA rose to 0.34 ng/mL, and an 18F-Fluciclovine scan was performed. The PET/CT and CT of the abdomen (*D*) demonstrated complete resolution of retroperitoneal metastatic lymph nodes. However, PET/CT, CT (*E, F*), and MIP (*G*) images demonstrated increased uptake within the left pubic bone and left external iliac lymph node, characteristic for residual disease (arrows).

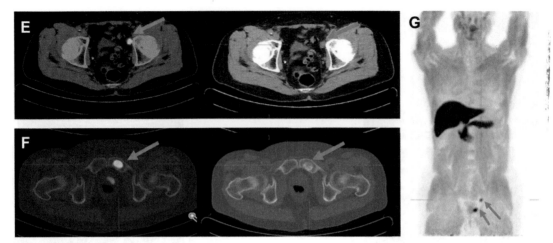

Fig. 6. (continued)

^{68}Ga-PSMA-11 has been reported to have a superior detection rate compared with ^{18}F-fluciclovine for extraprostatic metastasis, such as nodal or bone involvement.[51,52] Yet, due to low bladder excretion, ^{18}F-fluciclovine may be superior to current FDA-approved PSMA radiotracers for detection of local recurrence adjacent to the bladder. Interestingly, interim analysis of data from the randomized EMPIRE-2 Trial (NCT03762759) reported overall higher detection rates with ^{18}F-fluciclovine compared with ^{68}Ga-PSMA-11 mostly due to superior detection of local recurrence despite the use of furosemide with ^{68}Ga-PSMA-11. However, no significant differences were found for extraprostatic detection, which is similar to the findings from Pernthaler and coworkers.[52,53] Differences in detection rates may be due in part to differences in patient cohorts and experience with the technical performance of the PET study and image interpretation.

We expect that PSMA imaging will become the dominant PET technique, though ^{18}F-fluciclovine will still be of value to best define local recurrence adjacent to the bladder and when PSMA is negative or equivocal, as up to 10% of prostate cancer lesions may not express PSMA. Of course, PSMA is a theranostic pairing for PSMA radioligand therapy, an advantage which ^{18}F-fluciclovine does not possess. Finally, flare is reported with PSMA radiotracers due to upregulation of PSMA with ADT. While requiring further study, it is possible ^{18}F-fluciclovine PET may provide benefit in evaluating the response to hormonal therapy (**Fig. 6**).[44]

SUMMARY

[18]F-Fluciclovine PET is approved for the evaluation of patients with suspected prostate cancer recurrence. ^{18}F-fluciclovine PET is highly specific for the localization of extraprostatic disease even with negative conventional images and low PSA and has been reported to influence patients' management and improve outcome. With the recent FDA approval of PSMA PET, ^{18}F-fluciclovine will likely be used as an adjunct modality in patients with suspected occult local recurrence and/or negative PSMA findings.

ABBREVIATION/GLOSSARY LIST (MOST IMPORTANT ABBREVIATIONS IN ARTICLE)

1. Anti-1-amino-3-[^{18}F]-fluorocyclobutane-1-carboxylic acid (^{18}F-fluciclovine) is a synthetic non-metabolized amino acid analogue PET tracer that was approved in 2016 by the Food and Drug Administration (FDA) for positron emission tomography (PET) imaging of men with suspected prostate cancer recurrence after initial treatment.
2. Various studies have demonstrated the utility of ^{18}F-fluciclovine PET in the initial staging of prostate cancer, especially high-risk disease, with patient-level sensitivities for nodal involvement ranging from 40% to 66.7%, and specificities of 81.0% to 100%
3. The high PPV for extraprostatic disease characterization is important since the most critical element in deciding the appropriate treatment pathway in BCR is determining if cancer is locally recurrent or is also extraprostatic.
4. The lower specificity for local detection seems to be due to nonspecific radiotracer uptake in inflammation or benign hypertrophy in the intact prostate setting similar to the lower specificity reported in primary disease.

5. The EMPIRE-1 trial was a 165-patient randomized controlled trial designed to compare conventional imaging versus ^{8}F-fluciclovine-PET/CT to guide salvage radiotherapy in post-postprostatectomy BCR with the primary endpoint being three-year failure free survival. In the study arm in which patients underwent ^{18}F-fluciclovine PET/CT in addition to conventional imaging, there was a significant improvement in failure-free survival at 3 years (75.5% vs 63.0; p=0.003) and more so at 4 years (75.5% versus 51.2%; p<0.001).

6. A 113 patient retrospective analysis, positivity rate stratified by PSA levels for the localization of extraprostatic disease in BCR with PSA (ng/ml) >0-<0.2, 0.2-<0.5, and 0.5-<1 to be 30% (7/23), 44% (22/50), and 33% (13/40), respectively

7. ADT does not significantly influence the detection of prostate cancer recurrence with ^{18}F-fluciclovine PET/CT

8. Due to the rapid kinetics of the radiotracer, it is recommended to start scanning at 4 min post-injection (3-5 min), starting from below the pelvis to the skull base.

9. Though sclerotic lesions also display radiotracer uptake, some indolent dense sclerotic lesions may have none or minimal activity

10. For detection of cancer in the prostate, adjunct use of MR and ^{18}F-fluciclovine PET may have additive value

11. Due to the fast kinetics of ^{18}F-fluciclovine, it is critical to have a PET/MR protocol that leverages the recommended acquisition protocol of this radiotracer, including starting PET acquisition within 3-5 minutes of injection and not using a prolonged acquisition time per bed position

12. Since ^{18}F-fluciclovine reflects amino acid transport which is not specific to prostate cancer, other benign and malignant neoplasia may have ^{18}F-fluciclovine uptake

13. The interpretation of ^{18}F-fluciclovine is performed with a visual comparison of tumor to background ratio, usually the bone marrow and blood pool

14. Each radiotracer probes different aspects of the biology of prostate cancer: ^{18}F-fluciclovine that of tumor metabolism as reflected in amino acid transport, and PSMA as reflected in receptor upregulation/expression

15. ^{18}F-fluciclovine PET is highly specific for the localization of extraprostatic disease even with negative conventional images and low PSA and has been reported to influence patients' management and improve outcome. With the recent FDA approval of PSMA PET, ^{18}F-fluciclovine will likely be used as an adjunct modality in patients with suspected occult local recurrence and/or negative PSMA findings

CLINICS CARE POINTS

- 18F-fluciclovine is a synthetic non-metabolized amino acid analogue PET tracer that was approved in 2016 by the Food and Drug Administration for positron emission tomography imaging of men with suspected prostate cancer recurrence after initial treatment.

- 18F-fluciclovine PET/CT demonstrated high sensitivities and lower specifies for local prostate/ bed recurrence detection. False positive results may be related to nonspecific radiotracer uptake in inflammation or benign hypertrophy in the intact prostate.

- For the localization of extraprostatic disease, 18F-fluciclovine PET/CT demonstrated a positive predictive value of 92.3%

- 18F-fluciclovine PET/CT was proven to affect management in patients with both positive and negative 18F-fluciclovine PET/CT scans.

- The use of ^{18}F-fluciclovine-PET/CT to guide salvage radiotherapy in post-postprostatectomy biochemical recurrence resulted in better progression-free survival than conventional imaging.

DISCLOSURE

B Savir-Baruch Blue Earth Diagnostics, Consultant and Grants funds GE healthcare consultant.D M. Schuster Consultant: Syncona; AIM Specialty Health; Global Medical Solutions Taiwan; Progenics Pharmaceuticals, Inc. Research: Participates through the Emory Office of Sponsored Projects in full compliance with Emory University sponsored research and conflict of interest regulations in sponsored grants including those funded or partially funded by Blue Earth Diagnostics, Ltd; Nihon MediPhysics Co, Ltd.; Telix Pharmaceuticals (US) Inc.; Advanced Accelerator Applications; FUJIFILM Pharmaceuticals U.S.A., Inc; Amgen Inc. Educational: School of Breast Oncology; PrecisCa.

REFERENCES

1. Axumin (fluciclovine F 18) injection, printed labeling. Available at: https://www.accessdata.fda.gov/drugsatfda_docs/nda/2016/208054Orig1s000Lbl.pdf.

2. Okudaira H, Shikano N, Nishii R, et al. Putative transport mechanism and intracellular fate of trans-1-amino-3-18F-fluorocyclobutanecarboxylic acid in human prostate cancer. J Nucl Med 2011;52(5):822–9.

3. Oka S, Okudaira H, Yoshida Y, et al. Transport mechanisms of trans-1-amino-3-fluoro[1-(14)C]cyclobutanecarboxylic acid in prostate cancer cells. Nucl Med Biol 2012;39(1):109–19.

4. Nye JA, Schuster DM, Yu W, et al. Biodistribution and radiation dosimetry of the synthetic nonmetabolized amino acid analogue anti-18F-FACBC in humans. J Nucl Med 2007;48(6):1017–20.

5. Lovrec P, Schuster DM, Wagner RH, et al. Characterizing and mitigating bladder radioactivity on (18)F-fluciclovine PET/CT. J Nucl Med Technol 2020;48(1):24–9.

6. Turkbey B, Mena E, Shih J, et al. Localized prostate cancer detection with 18F FACBC PET/CT: comparison with MR imaging and histopathologic analysis. Radiology 2014;270(3):849–56.

7. Schuster DM, Taleghani PA, Nieh PT, et al. Characterization of primary prostate carcinoma by anti-1-amino-2-[(18)F]   -fluorocyclobutane-1-carboxylic acid (anti-3-[(18)F] FACBC) uptake. Am J Nucl Med Mol Imaging 2013;3(1):85–96.

8. Elschot M, Selnæs KM, Sandsmark E, et al. A PET/MRI study towards finding the optimal [(18)F]Fluciclovine PET protocol for detection and characterisation of primary prostate cancer. Eur J Nucl Med Mol Imaging 2017;44(4):695–703.

9. Jambor I, Kuisma A, Kahkonen E, et al. Prospective evaluation of (18)F-FACBC PET/CT and PET/MRI versus multiparametric MRI in intermediate-to high-risk prostate cancer patients (FLUCIPRO trial). Eur J Nucl Med Mol Imaging 2018;45(3):355–64.

10. Biscontini G, Romagnolo C, Cottignoli C, et al. 18F-Fluciclovine positron emission tomography in prostate cancer: a systematic review and diagnostic meta-analysis. Diagnostics (Basel, Switzerland) 2021;11(2):304.

11. Suzuki H, Jinnouchi S, Kaji Y, et al. Diagnostic performance of 18F-fluciclovine PET/CT for regional lymph node metastases in patients with primary prostate cancer: a multicenter phase II clinical trial. Jpn J Clin Oncol 2019;49(9):803–11.

12. Selnaes KM, Kruger-Stokke B, Elschot M, et al. (18)F-Fluciclovine PET/MRI for preoperative lymph node staging in high-risk prostate cancer patients. Eur Radiol 2018;28(8):3151–9.

13. Alemozaffar M, Akintayo AA, Abiodun-Ojo OA, et al. [(18)F]Fluciclovine positron emission tomography/computerized tomography for preoperative staging in patients with intermediate to high risk primary prostate cancer. J Urol 2020;204(4):734–40.

14. Hoekstra RJ, Beulens A, Vrijhof E, et al. Diagnostic accuracy of 18F-fluciclovine PET/CT in primary lymph node staging of prostate cancer. Nucl Med Commun 2021;42(5):476–81.

15. Zanoni L, Bianchi L, Nanni C, et al. [(18)F]-Fluciclovine PET/CT for preoperative nodal staging in high-risk primary prostate cancer: final results of a prospective trial. Eur J Nucl Med Mol Imaging 2021;49(1):390–409.

16. Schuster D, Votaw J, Nieh P, et al. Initial experience with the radiotracer anti-1-amino-3-F-18-fluorocyclobutane-1-carboxylic acid with PET/CT in prostate carcinoma. J Nucl Med 2007;48(1):56–63.

17. Schuster DM, Nieh PT, Jani AB, et al. Anti-3-[(18)F] FACBC positron emission tomography-computerized tomography and (111)In-capromab pendetide single photon emission computerized tomography-computerized tomography for recurrent prostate carcinoma: results of a prospective clinical trial. J Urol 2014;191(5):1446–53.

18. Odewole OA, Tade FI, Nieh PT, et al. Recurrent prostate cancer detection with anti-3-[18F]FACBC PET/CT: comparison with CT. Eur J Nucl Med Mol Imaging 2016;43(10):1773–83.

19. Andriole GL, Kostakoglu L, Chau A, et al. The impact of positron emission tomography with 18F-fluciclovine on the treatment of biochemical recurrence of prostate cancer: results from the LOCATE trial. J Urol 2019;201(2):322–31.

20. Abiodun-Ojo OA, Jani AB, Akintayo AA, et al. Salvage radiotherapy management decisions in postprostatectomy patients with recurrent prostate cancer based on (18)F-fluciclovine PET/CT guidance. J Nucl Med 2021;62(8):1089–96.

21. Chen B, Wei P, Macapinlac HA, et al. Comparison of 18F-Fluciclovine PET/CT and 99mTc-MDP bone scan in detection of bone metastasis in prostate cancer. Nucl Med Commun 2019;40(9):940–6.

22. Kim SJ, Lee SW. The role of 18F-fluciclovine PET in the management of prostate cancer: a systematic review and meta-analysis. Clin Radiol 2019;74(11):886–92.

23. Bach-Gansmo T, Nanni C, Nieh PT, et al. Multisite experience of the safety, detection rate and diagnostic performance of fluciclovine (18F) positron emission tomography/computerized tomography imaging in the staging of biochemically recurrent prostate cancer. J Urol 2017;197(3 Pt 1):676–83.

24. Abiodun-Ojo OA, Akintayo AA, Akin-Akintayo OO, et al. (18)F-fluciclovine parameters on targeted prostate biopsy associated with true positivity in recurrent prostate cancer. J Nucl Med 2019;60(11):1531–6.

25. Salavati A, Gencturk M, Koksel Y, et al. A bicentric retrospective analysis of clinical utility of (18)F-fluciclovine PET in biochemically recurrent prostate cancer following primary radiation therapy: is it helpful in

patients with a PSA rise less than the Phoenix criteria? Eur J Nucl Med Mol Imaging 2021;48(13): 4463–71.

26. Jani AB, Schreibmann E, Goyal S, et al. 18)F-flu-ciclovine-PET/CT imaging versus conventional imaging alone to guide postprostatectomy salvage radiotherapy for prostate cancer (EMPIRE-1): a single centre, open-label, phase 2/3 randomised controlled trial. Lancet 2021;397(10288): 1895–904.

27. Savir-Baruch B, Lovrec P, Solanki AA, et al. Fluorine-18-Labeled fluciclovine PET/CT in clinical practice: factors affecting the rate of detection of recurrent prostate cancer. AJR Am J Roentgenol 2019; 213(4):851–8.

28. Nakamoto R, Harrison C, Song H, et al. The clinical utility of (18)F-fluciclovine PET/CT in biochemically recurrent prostate cancer: an academic center experience post FDA approval. Mol Imaging Biol 2021;23(4):614–23.

29. Bulbul JE, Grybowski D, Lovrec P, et al. Positivity rate of [(18)F]fluciclovine PET/CT in patients with suspected prostate cancer recurrence at PSA levels below 1 ng/mL. Mol Imaging Biol : MIB : official Publ Acad Mol Imaging 2022;24(1):42–9.

30. Marcus C, Abiodun-Ojo OA, Jani AB, et al. Clinical utility of (18)F-Fluciclovine PET/CT in recurrent prostate cancer with very low (≤0.3 ng/mL) prostate-specific antigen levels. Am J Nucl Med Mol Imaging 2021;11(5):406–14.

31. Bulbul J.E., Hashem A., Grybowski D., et al., Effect of hormonal therapy on ¹⁸F-fluciclovine PET/CT in thedetection of prostate cancer recurrence, localization of metastatic disease, and correlation with prostate-specific antigen, Urol Oncol, 40 (8), 2022, 379.e9-379.e16.

32. Savir-Baruch B, Choyke PL, Rowe SP, et al. Role of (18)F-fluciclovine and prostate-specific membrane antigen PET/CT in guiding management of oligometastatic prostate cancer: AJR expert panel narrative review. AJR Am J Roentgenol 2021;216(4):851–9.

33. Kim EH, Siegel BA, Teoh EJ, et al. Prostate cancer recurrence in patients with negative or equivocal conventional imaging: a role for (18)F-fluciclovine-PET/CT in delineating sites of recurrence and identifying patients with oligometastatic disease. Urol Oncol 2021;39(6):365–9.

34. Savir-Baruch B, Banks KP, McConathy JE, et al. ACR-ACNM practice parameter for the performance of fluorine-18 fluciclovine-PET/CT for recurrent prostate cancer. Clin Nucl Med 2018;43(12):909–17.

35. Tade FI, Sajdak RA, Gabriel M, et al. Best practices for (18)F-fluciclovine PET/CT imaging of recurrent prostate cancer: a guide for technologists. J Nucl Med Technol 2019;47(4):282–7.

36. Nanni C, Zanoni L, Bach-Gansmo T, et al. [(18)F]Flu-ciclovine PET/CT: joint EANM and SNMMI procedure guideline for prostate cancer imaging-version 1.0. Eur J Nucl Med Mol Imaging 2020;47(3):579–91.

37. Gill HS, Tade F, Greenwald DT, et al. Metastatic male breast cancer with increased uptake on 18F-fluciclo-vine PET/CT scan. Clin Nucl Med 2018;43(1):23–4.

38. Schuster DM, Nanni C, Fanti S, et al. Anti-1-amino-3-18F-fluorocyclobutane-1-carboxylic acid: physiologic uptake patterns, incidental findings, and variants that may simulate disease. J Nucl Med : official Publ Soc Nucl Med 2014;55(12):1986–92.

39. Bitar R, Martiniova L, Bell D, et al. Incidental 18F-Fluciclovine uptake in a warthin tumor of the parotid gland in a patient undergoing PET/CT imaging for biochemical recurrent prostate cancer. Clin Nucl Med 2020;45(4):e208–10.

40. Raghavan K, Flavell RR, Westphalen AC, et al. Gastrointestinal stromal tumor incidentally detected on 18F-Fluciclovine PET/CT. Clin Nucl Med 2021; 46(4):345–7.

41. Parihar AS, Schmidt LR, Dehdashti F, et al. Detection of additional primary neoplasms on (18)F-Fluciclo-vine PET/CT in patients with primary prostate cancer. J Nucl Med 2021;63(5):713–9.

42. Hoyle JM, Lenzie A, Galgano SJ, et al. Synchronous malignancies identified by (18)F-fluciclovine positron emission tomography for prostate cancer: case series and mini-review. Clin Genitourin Cancer 2021;19(1):e37–40.

43. Elschot M, Selnaes KM, Sandsmark E, et al. Combined (18)F-fluciclovine PET/MRI shows potential for detection and characterization of high-risk prostate cancer. J Nucl Med : official Publ Soc Nucl Med 2018;59(5):762–8.

44. Galgano SJ, McDonald AM, Rais-Bahrami S, et al. Utility of (18)F-fluciclovine PET/MRI for staging newly diagnosed high-risk prostate cancer and evaluating response to initial androgen deprivation therapy: a prospective single-arm pilot study. AJR Am J Roentgenol 2021;217(3):720–9.

45. Selnæs KM, Krüger-Stokke B, Elschot M, et al. Detection of recurrent prostate cancer with 18F-fluci-clovine PET/MRI. Front Oncol 2020;10(2930).

46. Chen B, Bathala TK, Xu G, et al. Comparison of diagnostic utility of fluciclovine PET/CT versus pelvic multiparametric MRI for prostate cancer in the pelvis in the setting of rising PSA after initial treatment. Clin Nucl Med 2020;45(5):349–55.

47. PYLARIFY® (piflufolastat F 18) injection, for intravenous use Initial U.S. Approval: 2021. Available at: https://www.accessdata.fda.gov/drugsatfda_docs/nda/2021/214793Orig1s000lbl.pdf.

48. Illuccix FDA approval press release. Available at: https://telixpharma.com/news-media/fda-approves-telixs-prostate-cancer-imaging-product-illuccix/.

49. Ga PSMA-11 UCLA/UCSF. Available at: https://www.accessdata.fda.gov/drugsatfda_docs/label/2020/212642s000lbl.pdf.

50. NCCN prostate 2. 2022. Available at: https://www.nccn.org/professionals/physician_gls/pdf/prostate.pdf.

51. Calais J, Ceci F, Eiber M, et al. 18)F-fluciclovine PET-CT and (68)Ga-PSMA-11 PET-CT in patients with early biochemical recurrence after prostatectomy: a prospective, single-centre, single-arm, comparative imaging trial. Lancet Oncol 2019;20(9):1286–94.

52. Pernthaler B, Kulnik R, Gstettner C, et al. A prospective head-to-head comparison of 18F-fluciclovine with 68Ga-PSMA-11 in biochemical recurrence of prostate cancer in PET/CT. Clin Nucl Med 2019;44(10):e566–73.

53. Abiodun-Ojo O, Jani A, Adediran O, et al. 18F-Fluciclovine PET/CT and 68Ga-PSMA PET/CT guidance of salvage radiotherapy in patients with biochemical recurrence postprostatectomy: interim analysis of a secondary endpoint from a randomized trial. Radiological Society of North America (RSNA) Scientific Assembly and Annual Meeting. Chicago, Illinois; 2021. RSNA meeting was in Nov 28, 2021 – Dec 2, 2021.

PET Imaging Using Gallium-68 (^{68}Ga) RM2

Heying Duan, MD, Andrei Iagaru, MD*

KEYWORDS

• ^{68}Ga-RM2 • GRPR • Bombesin • PET • Prostate cancer

KEY POINTS

- Gastrin-releasing peptide receptors (GRPR) are overexpressed in prostate cancer.
- Gallium-68 (^{68}Ga) RM2 is a synthetic GRPR antagonist that has high GRPR affinity with a favorable biodistribution and dosimetry, which can be used for both imaging and therapy in patients with prostate cancer.
- ^{68}Ga-RM2 and prostate-specific membrane antigen show discordant uptake patterns at initial diagnosis and biochemical recurrence of prostate cancer which suggests that both might be complementary to each other.

INTRODUCTION

One in every six to eight men will be diagnosed with prostate cancer (PC) during their lifetime.[1] PC is the second most frequent non-cutaneous cancer in men with an estimated 1.4 million new cases and 375,000 deaths ranking as the fifth leading cause of cancer deaths among men in 2020 worldwide.[2] Early and accurate detection of suspected PC or biochemical recurrence (BCR) is critical to ensure adequate and timely patient management. The tumor biology of PC is heterogenous ranging from indolent disease (Gleason score 6) to clinically significant cancers (Gleason score $\geq$7). Even in significant cancers, some progress and metastasize more rapidly than others. Therefore, it is important to distinguish between patients with nonaggressive tumors, which will benefit from active surveillance, and those with clinically significant cancers, which will require subsequent treatment.

The role of imaging for staging and restaging of PC is advancing at a rapid pace. The use of PET combined with computed tomography (CT) or MRI has become indispensable as it provides the best of two worlds, anatomical and biological information. PET/MRI with its high soft-tissue contrast enhances imaging of local disease. Modern PET scanners equipped with highly sensitive detectors based on silicon photomultipliers and using new reconstruction algorithms improve image quality.[3] Not only is technology advancing but so are imaging agents targeting different receptors on the PC cell. The most widely used radiopharmaceuticals target the prostate-specific membrane antigen (PSMA). PSMA is overexpressed in 90% of PC and PSMA-labeled compounds can be used for theragnostic, ie, targeted molecular imaging with subsequent radionuclide treatment. This concept of *to see what you treat and to treat what you see* enables personalized treatment selection, planning, and evaluation with one single agent and has revolutionized the landscape of PC imaging and treatment.[4–7] However, to borrow a phrase from William Shakespeare, *all that glitters is not gold*, the one perfect radiotracer to image all clinical scenarios of PC does not exist. Despite its name, PSMA is also expressed by various benign and inflammatory tissues,[8,9] and other malignancies, leading to false-positive findings.[10–16] Up to 10% of prostate adenocarcinomas and neuroendocrine differentiated PC cells[17] do not express PSMA.[18] Therefore, there is a need for other targets for PC imaging.

Division of Nuclear Medicine and Molecular Imaging, Department of Radiology, Stanford University, 300 Pasteur Drive, H2200, Stanford, CA 94305, USA
* Corresponding author.
E-mail address: aiagaru@stanford.edu

PET Clin 17 (2022) 621–629
https://doi.org/10.1016/j.cpet.2022.07.006
1556-8598/22/© 2022 Elsevier Inc. All rights reserved.

Gastrin-releasing peptide receptors (GRPR) are highly overexpressed in several cancers such as PC,[19–22] breast cancer,[23,24] small cell lung cancer,[25] gastrointestinal stromal, and neuroendocrine tumors.[26,27] Although PC cells show a high density of GRPR, benign lesions such as benign prostatic hyperplasia and prostatitis show less expression.[19,21,28] In metastatic disease, 86% of lymph nodes and 53% of bone metastases overexpress GRPR.[21,29] These characteristics make GRPR an optimal target for imaging and treatment.

In this review article, we briefly discuss the background of GRPR and its antagonist RM2 and focus on recent advances in PET imaging with gallium-68 (^{68}Ga) radiolabeled RM2 for PC at initial staging and BCR. Finally, we give an outlook into future directions with GRPR antagonists.

GASTRIN-RELEASING PEPTIDE AND GASTRIN-RELEASING PEPTIDE RECEPTOR

GRPR is a peptide receptor of the bombesin (BBN) family. The name is related to the first isolation of the amphibian neuropeptide BBN from the skin of the European fire-bellied toad *Bombina bombina*. The mammalian BBN was named after its main function, gastrin-releasing peptide (GRP) and neuromedin-B (NMB). Their biological actions are regulated by three G-protein coupled receptors: BB_1-R (NMB receptor), BB_2-R (GRPR), and BB_3-R (orphan receptor); for the latter no ligand was found so far.[30]

GRP regulates multiple physiological processes of cellular growth, function, and intercellular communication as they act as neurotransmitters, secrete hormones, modulate the immune response by releasing chemokines and cytokines, and most importantly for cancer development, growth factors.[21] These autocrine growth factors stimulate tumor proliferation and differentiation with consecutive overexpression of GRPR.[31–33] The mitogenic effect of GRP could lead to the assumption that GRPR is closely related to malignant cell transformation. Some studies[34,35] support this hypothesis including a study where a positive correlation between ^{68}Ga-RM2 uptake and prostate-specific antigen (PSA) velocity was seen in BCR of PC.[36] Other studies, however, show that the lower the Gleason score and PSA value, and the smaller the tumor size, the higher the expression of GRPR.[19,20,37] Larger, prospective trials with correlation to histopathology at various different stages of PC are needed to resolve this controversy.

GASTRIN-RELEASING PEPTIDE RECEPTOR AGONISTS VERSUS ANTAGONISTS

Initially, GRPR agonists were explored as the receptor/ligand complex gets internalized into the cell resulting in a prolonged intracellular retention and subsequent tracer accumulation. However, once the peptide binds to GRPR, the activated receptor sets a complex cellular cascade in motion that includes activating second messengers resulting in gastrointestinal side effects such as nausea, abdominal cramps, and diarrhea.[38] Similar to somatostatin receptors where antagonists have been found to bind to their specific receptor subtype significantly greater than the agonist,[39] the focus shifted toward GRPR antagonists. As it turned out, there are even more receptors per cell available for GRPR antagonists than for agonists. The reason why is that with agonists, not only does the receptor/ligand complex get internalized, but also the surrounding GRPR leaving overall lesser GRPR on the cell surface to bind to.[40,41] Imaging with GRPR antagonists resulted in a better tumor-to-normal tissue ratio and no gastrointestinal adverse effects as there is no activation of the cell signaling cascade.[42]

The synthesis of peptides is fairly straightforward and producing large quantities is easily feasible. GRPR antagonists show rapid tissue penetration in vivo, fast blood clearance because of small size, and low antigenicity.[43] However, peptides are often metabolically unstable. Efforts were underway to improve metabolic stability and pharmacokinetic performance by introducing different chelators and linkers in the amino acid sequence. RM2 is the most widely used synthetic GRPR antagonist. DOTA is used as a chelator to radiolabel RM2 to ^{68}Ga for PET imaging. This conjugation creates stable complexes, which allows for an easy kit production. ^{68}Ga-RM2 shows high selective binding affinity to GRPR, metabolic stability, and prolonged retention in lesions.[44]

BIODISTRIBUTION AND DOSIMETRY

The biodistribution of ^{68}Ga-RM2 shows an excretion almost exclusively through the urinary tract, without binding to the renal cortex. Intense uptake is noted in the pancreas as GRP is regulating enteropancreatic hormone release. However, only mild uptake is seen in the liver and gastrointestinal tract. This combined with the rapid blood clearance and renal washout contributes to a reduction of background uptake. This biodistribution pattern is advantageous for the detection of liver metastases and abdominal and pelvic lymph node metastases, which might have been otherwise masked by bowel uptake. No significant uptake is seen in the brain, salivary glands, myocardium, lungs, liver, spleen, adrenal glands, skeleton, muscle, and fat.[45]

Concordant with biodistribution, dosimetry shows the highest absorbed dose in the urinary bladder wall and pancreas followed by the kidneys.[46,47] In contrast to GRPR agonists,[48,49] a rapid organ clearance, especially from the pancreas, is noted but not in the tumor, resulting in a high tumor to background ratio.[44]

In summary, ⁶⁸Ga-RM2 has an excellent biosafety profile, favorable pharmacokinetics, low radiation dose, and selective and high binding affinity to GRPR with rapid organ and blood clearance which are also advantageous characteristics for theragnostic purposes.[44,50,51]

GALLIUM-68 (⁶⁸GA) RM2 AT INITIAL STAGING

Early detection and diagnosis of PC present a challenge as PSA screening has dramatically increased the detection of mostly low-grade PC. The overdiagnosis and overtreatment of clinically nonsignificant PC was not only related to an increase in therapy-associated adverse events such as erectile dysfunction and incontinence but also incurred a significant economic burden on the health care system. As a result, the US Preventive Services Task Force considered PSA screening to have an unfavorable risk–benefit analysis where the harms outweighed the benefits and recommended against routine PSA screening.[52] The challenge is to distinguish these indolent cancers from clinically significant PC who will require treatment. As a next step, it is also critical to further stratify aggressive PC into localized and metastasized diseases as this defines patient management and treatment selection.

Molecular imaging is a fast, noninvasive, and safe method to image the whole body to diagnose and localize suspected PC. The American Society of Clinical Oncology recommends imaging for all patients with unfavorable intermediate- or high-risk PC[53] and specifically endorsed PET imaging in men with a high risk of metastatic disease or rising PSA after prostatectomy when anatomical imaging and bone scintigraphy are negative or equivocal.[54] GRPR has been reported to be particularly overexpressed in earlier stages of PC, making it a promising target at initial diagnosis.[19]

⁶⁸Ga-RM2 was first investigated by Kähkönen and colleagues. They evaluated 11 men with newly diagnosed PC and 3 with BCR. For detection of primary PC, the group found high sensitivity, specificity, and accuracy at 89%, 81%, and 83%, respectively. Compared with whole-mount prostatectomy histology, all true positive lesions interestingly correlated to significant PC with Gleason score ≥7, contrary to what was reported before in in vitro studies.[19,20] False-positive intraprostatic lesions were found to be benign prostatic hyperplasia.[42] Similar results were seen in another prospective study where additionally no correlation of ⁶⁸Ga-RM2 with Gleason score was found.[55] These findings might be attributed to different binding mechanisms at the GRPR in vivo which requires the presence of the receptor on the cell surface, and in vitro immunohistochemistry with GRPR antibodies where the presence of GRPR on the cell surface is not necessary. Immunohistochemical staining for GRPR and PSMA found a weaker staining of GRPR compared with PSMA, whereas their respective expression was not correlated. This suggests that GRPR and PSMA expression are unrelated, but might complement each other.[55] A study in patients with biopsy-proven PC undergoing PET/CT with both ⁶⁸Ga-RM2 and ⁶⁸Ga-PSMA11 support this theory as ⁶⁸Ga-RM2 and ⁶⁸Ga-PSMA11 showed an inverse uptake pattern.[56]

A recently published study in men with biopsy-proven, high-risk PC who underwent ⁶⁸Ga-PSMA11 (n = 22) and ⁶⁸Ga-RM2 PET/MRI (n = 19) for staging found that the primary PC was detected by all modalities, whereas ⁶⁸Ga-RM2 was negative in one patient. MRI was superior at detecting seminal vesicle involvement on MRI, where ⁶⁸Ga-RM2 was negative in these patients. ⁶⁸Ga-PSMA11 detected more lymph and bone metastases compared with ⁶⁸Ga-RM2 and MRI.[57] These results again show a heterogenous expression of GRPR and PSMA. Our group evaluated 41 men pre-prostatectomy with ⁶⁸Ga-RM2 of which 17 had additional ⁶⁸Ga-PSMA11 PET.⁶⁸Ga-RM2 showed a detection rate of 93% for intraprostatic PC lesions. Uptake in lymph nodes was lower than in PC lesions; however, 16/19 subcentimeter pelvic lymph nodes were histopathologically verified and follow-up imaging confirmed another two lymph node metastases. ⁶⁸Ga-RM2 positively correlated with PSA, suggesting that ⁶⁸Ga-RM2 PET might be better suited for the staging of high-risk patients. Concordant with a prior study, ⁶⁸Ga-RM2 and ⁶⁸Ga-PSMA11 were poorly correlated not only in localization but also in intensity as **Fig. 1** illustrates.[58]

GALLIUM-68 (⁶⁸GA) RM2 AT RESTAGING AND BIOCHEMICAL RECURRENCE

After radical prostatectomy, PSA decreases to undetectable levels and even a slight rise of ≥0.2 ng/

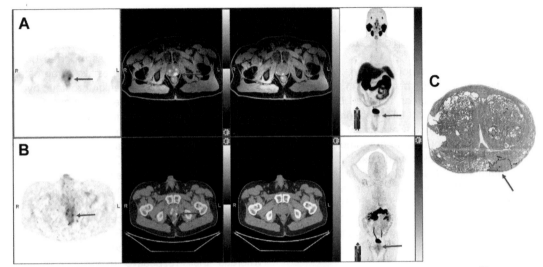

Fig. 1. A 65-year-old patient with high-risk, clinical stage T2a PC and presurgical PSA of 3.80 ng/mL. ^{68}Ga-PSMA11 PET/MRI (*A*), axial PET, fused PET/MRI, MRI, and MIP images, respectively) and ^{68}Ga-RM2 PET/CT (*B*), axial PET, fused PET/CT, CT, and MIP images, respectively) both show true positive focal uptake left posterior (*arrows*), however, of different intensity. Histopathology (*C*) revealed a corresponding Gleason score 4 + 3 prostate adenocarcinoma left posterior (*arrow*).

mL with a second confirmatory PSA of at least 0.2 ng/mL indicates BCR.[59] After definitive treatment with radiation therapy however, PSA reaches a nadir and BCR is defined as rise of ≥2 ng/mL above nadir.[60] BCR has been reported to be more likely to occur within the first five years of initial treatment.[61] Although PSA is pivotal in indicating the recurrence of disease, it does not reflect its location. Early identification of the site of relapse defines subsequent patient management and may prevent potentially futile and harmful treatments. However, at early BCR, when low PSA levels indicate low disease volume, anatomical imaging and bone scintigraphy often fail to depict the localization of BCR. PET has a better diagnostic performance and helps to map the knowledge gap. Furthermore, PET can also stratify according to the extent of the disease resulting in better treatment strategies which in turn affects prognosis. In a meta-analysis, ^{68}Ga-PSMA11 PET showed best detection rates of >70% when PSA is > 1 ng/mL and further with decreasing PSA (50% for 0.2–0.49 ng/mL, and 34% for <0.2 ng/mL).[62] Imaging with GRPR antagonists plays a particular important role in these PSMA-negative patients.

In a prospective study evaluating 32 men with BCR and negative anatomical imaging and bone scintigraphy, ^{68}Ga-RM2 showed a high detection rate of 71% for recurrent disease whereas simultaneous MRI was only at 34%. A positive correlation was seen between ^{68}Ga-RM2 positivity and PSA velocity, which might indicate that PSA velocity could predict RM2 positivity and conversely, a

negative ^{68}Ga-RM2 PET might suggest a more favorable prognosis.[36] Larger studies are needed to underpin this theory.

The hitherto largest study investigating GRPR- and PSMA-targeted imaging for BCR compared ^{68}Ga-RM2 PET/MRI (*n* = 50) to ^{68}Ga-PSMA11 (*n* = 23) or the F-18 (^{18}F) labeled DCFPyL (*n* = 27) PET/CT. ^{68}Ga-RM2 and ^{68}Ga-PSMA11/^{18}F-DCFPyL showed similar positivity rates; however, discordant uptake was observed in 18 patients (**Fig. 2**). No correlation was found for PSA or PSA velocity.[63]

An incongruent uptake pattern was observed when ^{68}Ga-RM2 was compared with ^{18}F-fluorocholine (^{18}F-ECH) in a small cohort of 16 BCR patients with negative or inconclusive ^{18}F-ECH PET/CT. ^{68}Ga-RM2 PET/CT identified local recurrent disease, lymph node, lung, and bone metastases in 63% of the patients of which the majority (70%) were confirmed by either histology, further imaging, or response to site-directed therapy. However, the time interval between both scans was quite long at 6 months and PSA progressed over time which is why PSA was significantly higher when the patients underwent ^{68}Ga-RM2 PET/CT.[64]

These studies all show that ^{68}Ga-RM2 PET is a valuable tool for men with BCR of PC especially when other molecular imaging is negative or equivocal. However, of note is that the expression of PSMA is affected by treatments targeting the androgen receptor pathway leading to an increased uptake, and both PSMA and GRPR are affected by taxane-based chemotherapy.[65,66] In

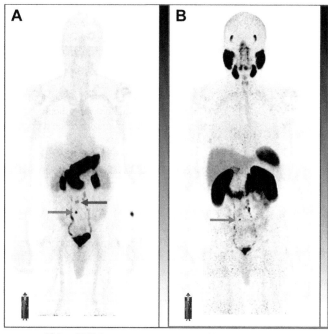

^{68}Ga-RM2   **^{68}Ga-PSMA11**

Fig. 2. Heterogenous expression pattern of PSMA and GRPR in a 70-year-old man with biochemical recurrent prostate cancer: ^{68}Ga-RM2 (*A*) shows uptake in multiple retroperitoneal lymph nodes (*red and blue arrows*), whereas ^{68}Ga-PSMA11 (*B*) PET was positive in only one lymph node (*blue arrow*).

the setting of BCR, it might be difficult to identify the optimal radiopharmaceutical for re-staging given the highly variable treatment histories that BCR patients have.

FUTURE PERSPECTIVES
Different Bombesin Analogs

Currently, efforts are underway to investigate different BBN analogs. As targeted, precision medicine is critical nowadays, BBN analogs which can be used for theragnostic are investigated. NeoBOMB1 is a novel DOTA-coupled GRPR antagonist which can be radiolabeled with ^{68}Ga for PET imaging or Lu-177 (^{177}Lu) for peptide receptor radionuclide therapy (PRRT). Preclinical and clinical studies showed promising results with high GRPR affinity, metabolic stability, high tumor retention, and favorable safety profile.[67–69] A study to compare ^{68}Ga-NeoBOMB1 to ^{68}Ga-PSMA R2 in men with BCR after initial definitive treatment is currently ongoing (NCT03698370).

Bispecific Heterodimers

The heterogenous expression of GRPR and PSMA throughout all stages of PC prompted research in the direction of bispecific heterodimers that can target both. Simultaneous targeting of GRPR and PSMA could therefore increase diagnostic accuracy and consecutively tailor a more efficient treatment strategy. Several compounds have been

developed and labeled with different radioisotopes for molecular imaging. Preclinical studies have shown promising results with a favorable biodistribution and rapid blood and organ clearance through the kidneys. High receptor affinity was seen, but not homogenously distributed between GRPR and PSMA.[70–73] However, the translation into clinics is highly anticipated.

Imaging Beyond Disease Staging

The diagnosis of PC is commonly made through prostate biopsy, guided by multiparametric MRI (mpMRI). However, up to 10% of PC may be missed by mpMRI. A study to investigate the usefulness of a combined approach of ^{68}Ga-RM2 and ^{68}Ga-PSMA PET/MRI is currently underway with promising preliminary results of PET identifying more clinically significant PC lesions than mpMRI (NCT03809078).

Another important area where molecular imaging can have a big impact is for therapy guidance and response evaluation of local treatments such as high-intensity focused ultrasound (HIFU) or high-dose rate (HDR) brachytherapy. This is currently investigated with again a combined approach of ^{68}Ga-RM2 and ^{68}Ga-PSMA PET/MRI by the same group. Preliminary results show that PET accurately identified the dominant intraprostatic lesion and verified response to treatment (NCT03949517).

SUMMARY

Molecular imaging is indispensable in the era of precision medicine. It visualizes tumor biology and can stratify responders to nonresponders for subsequent PRRT. In that manner, the emphasis on PC is to identify clinically significant cancers from indolent disease. The heterogeneity of GRPR and PSMA expression in primary and metastatic PC has been shown in multiple studies. More prospective trials with larger cohorts using GRPR antagonists are needed, especially in comparison to the currently most widely used ^{68}Ga-PSMA11, to better understand their relationship and potential predictive value of tumor biology and aggressiveness in different types and stages of PC. However, we also need to shed light on how standard of care treatments can impact receptor expression and conversely whether an increase or decrease of receptor expression can be induced by certain treatments. This could shift the susceptibility of PRRT.

CLINICS CARE POINTS

- Gallium-68 (^{68}Ga) RM2 PET has high sensitivity, specificity, and accuracy at initial staging and restaging at biochemical recurrence for prostate cancer.
- ^{68}Ga-RM2 PET might be better suited to image high-risk PC at initial staging.
- ^{68}Ga-RM2 and ^{68}Ga-PSMA11/^{18}F DCFPyL express a heterogenous expression pattern that reflects the heterogeneity of tumor biology in prostate cancer.
- Simultaneous targeting of gastrin-releasing peptide receptor and prostate-specific membrane antigen with bispecific radiopharmaceuticals could improve diagnostic sensitivity and specificity and are currently investigated.
- ^{68}Ga-RM2 PET accurately detects the dominant lesion for biopsy guidance and local intraprostatic treatment, and is valuable in the evaluation of treatment response.

DISCLOSURE

The authors have nothing to disclose.

REFERENCES

1. Schroder FH, Hugosson J, Roobol MJ, et al. Prostate-cancer mortality at 11 years of follow-up. N Engl J Med 2012;366(11):981–90.
2. Sung H, Ferlay J, Siegel RL, et al. Global cancer statistics 2020: GLOBOCAN estimates of incidence and mortality worldwide for 36 cancers in 185 countries. CA Cancer J Clin 2021;71(3):209–49.
3. Baratto L, Duan H, Ferri V, et al. The effect of various beta values on image quality and semiquantitative measurements in 68Ga-RM2 and 68Ga-PSMA-11 PET/MRI images reconstructed with a block sequential regularized expectation maximization algorithm. Clin Nucl Med 2020;45(7):506–13.
4. Fendler WP, Ferdinandus J, Czernin J, et al. Impact of (68)Ga-PSMA-11 PET on the management of recurrent prostate cancer in a prospective single-arm clinical trial. J Nucl Med 2020;61(12):1793–9.
5. Sonni I, Eiber M, Fendler WP, et al. Impact of (68)Ga-PSMA-11 PET/CT on staging and management of prostate cancer patients in various clinical settings: a prospective single-center study. J Nucl Med 2020;61(8):1153–60.
6. Dietlein M, Kobe C, Kuhnert G, et al. Comparison of [(18)F]DCFPyL and [(68)Ga]Ga-PSMA-HBED-CC for PSMA-PET imaging in patients with relapsed prostate cancer. Mol Imaging Biol 2015;17(4):575–84.
7. Rasul S, Hacker M, Kretschmer-Chott E, et al. Clinical outcome of standardized (177)Lu-PSMA-617 therapy in metastatic prostate cancer patients receiving 7400 MBq every 4 weeks. Eur J Nucl Med Mol Imaging 2020;47(3):713–20.
8. Sathekge M, Lengana T, Modiselle M, et al. 68Ga-PSMA-HBED-CC PET imaging in breast carcinoma patients. Eur J Nucl Med Mol Imaging 2017;44(4):689–94.
9. Rhee H, Blazak J, Tham CM, et al. Pilot study: use of gallium-68 PSMA PET for detection of metastatic lesions in patients with renal tumour. EJNMMI Res 2016;6(1):76.
10. Sasikumar A, Joy A, Nanabala R, et al. 68Ga-PSMA PET/CT false-positive tracer uptake in paget disease. Clin Nucl Med 2016;41(10):e454–5.
11. Noto B, Vrachimis A, Schafers M, et al. Subacute stroke mimicking cerebral metastasis in 68Ga-PSMA-HBED-CC PET/CT. Clin Nucl Med 2016;41(10):e449–51.
12. Hermann RM, Djannatian M, Czech N, et al. Prostate-specific membrane antigen PET/CT: false-positive results due to sarcoidosis? Case Rep Oncol 2016;9(2):457–63.
13. Rowe SP, Gorin MA, Hammers HJ, et al. Imaging of metastatic clear cell renal cell carcinoma with PSMA-targeted (1)(8)F-DCFPyL PET/CT. Ann Nucl Med 2015;29(10):877–82.
14. Verburg FA, Krohn T, Heinzel A, et al. First evidence of PSMA expression in differentiated thyroid cancer using [(6)(8)Ga]PSMA-HBED-CC PET/CT. Eur J Nucl Med Mol Imaging 2015;42(10):1622–3.

15. Schwenck J, Tabatabai G, Skardelly M, et al. In vivo visualization of prostate-specific membrane antigen in glioblastoma. Eur J Nucl Med Mol Imaging 2015; 42(1):170–1.
16. Krohn T, Verburg FA, Pufe T, et al. [(68)Ga]PSMA-HBED uptake mimicking lymph node metastasis in coeliac ganglia: an important pitfall in clinical practice. Eur J Nucl Med Mol Imaging 2015;42(2):210–4.
17. Tosoian JJ, Gorin MA, Rowe SP, et al. Correlation of PSMA-Targeted (18)F-DCFPyL PET/CT findings with immunohistochemical and genomic data in a patient with metastatic neuroendocrine prostate cancer. Clin Genitourin Cancer 2017;15(1):e65–8.
18. Maurer T, Gschwend JE, Rauscher I, et al. Diagnostic efficacy of (68)Gallium-PSMA positron emission tomography compared to conventional imaging for lymph node staging of 130 consecutive patients with intermediate to high risk prostate cancer. J Urol 2016;195(5):1436–43.
19. Korner M, Waser B, Rehmann R, et al. Early overexpression of GRP receptors in prostatic carcinogenesis. Prostate 2014;74(2):217–24.
20. Beer M, Montani M, Gerhardt J, et al. Profiling gastrin-releasing peptide receptor in prostate tissues: clinical implications and molecular correlates. Prostate 2012;72(3):318–25.
21. Markwalder R, Reubi JC. Gastrin-releasing peptide receptors in the human prostate: relation to neoplastic transformation. Cancer Res 1999;59(5):1152–9.
22. Wieser G, Mansi R, Grosu AL, et al. Positron emission tomography (PET) imaging of prostate cancer with a gastrin releasing peptide receptor antagonist–from mice to men. Theranostics 2014;4(4):412–9.
23. Stoykow C, Erbes T, Maecke HR, et al. Gastrin-releasing peptide receptor imaging in breast cancer using the receptor antagonist (68)Ga-RM2 and PET. Theranostics 2016;6(10):1641–50.
24. Dalm SU, Martens JW, Sieuwerts AM, et al. In vitro and in vivo application of radiolabeled gastrin-releasing peptide receptor ligands in breast cancer. J Nucl Med 2015;56(5):752–7.
25. Mattei J, Achcar RD, Cano CH, et al. Gastrin-releasing peptide receptor expression in lung cancer. Arch Pathol Lab Med 2014;138(1):98–104.
26. Reubi JC, Korner M, Waser B, et al. High expression of peptide receptors as a novel target in gastrointestinal stromal tumours. Eur J Nucl Med Mol Imaging 2004;31(6):803–10.
27. Reubi JC. Peptide receptor expression in GEP-NET. Virchows Arch 2007;451(Suppl 1):S47–50.
28. Accardo A, Galli F, Mansi R, et al. Pre-clinical evaluation of eight DOTA coupled gastrin-releasing peptide receptor (GRP-R) ligands for in vivo targeting of receptor-expressing tumors. EJNMMI Res 2016; 6(1):17.
29. Ananias HJ, van den Heuvel MC, Helfrich W, et al. Expression of the gastrin-releasing peptide receptor, the prostate stem cell antigen and the prostate-specific membrane antigen in lymph node and bone metastases of prostate cancer. Prostate 2009;69(10):1101–8.
30. Jensen RT, Battey JF, Spindel ER, et al. International Union of Pharmacology. LXVIII. Mammalian bombesin receptors: nomenclature, distribution, pharmacology, signaling, and functions in normal and disease states. Pharmacol Rev 2008;60(1):1–42.
31. Schroeder RP, de Visser M, van Weerden WM, et al. Androgen-regulated gastrin-releasing peptide receptor expression in androgen-dependent human prostate tumor xenografts. Int J Cancer 2010; 126(12):2826–34.
32. Xiao C, Reitman ML. Bombesin-like receptor 3: physiology of a functional orphan. Trends Endocrinol Metab 2016;27(9):603–5.
33. Varasteh Z, Aberg O, Velikyan I, et al. In vitro and in vivo evaluation of a (18)F-labeled high affinity NOTA conjugated bombesin antagonist as a PET ligand for GRPR-targeted tumor imaging. PLoS One 2013;8(12):e81932.
34. Nagasaki S, Nakamura Y, Maekawa T, et al. Immunohistochemical analysis of gastrin-releasing peptide receptor (GRPR) and possible regulation by estrogen receptor betacx in human prostate carcinoma. Neoplasma 2012;59(2):224–32.
35. Constantinides C, Lazaris AC, Haritopoulos KN, et al. Immunohistochemical detection of gastrin releasing peptide in patients with prostate cancer. World J Urol 2003;21(3):183–7.
36. Minamimoto R, Sonni I, Hancock S, et al. Prospective evaluation of (68)Ga-RM2 PET/MRI in patients with biochemical recurrence of prostate cancer and negative findings on conventional imaging. J Nucl Med 2018;59(5):803–8.
37. Schollhammer R, De Clermont Gallerande H, Yacoub M, et al. Comparison of the radiolabeled PSMA-inhibitor (111)In-PSMA-617 and the radiolabeled GRP-R antagonist (111)In-RM2 in primary prostate cancer samples. EJNMMI Res 2019;9(1):52.
38. Bertaccini G, Impicciatore M. Action of bombesin on the motility of the stomach. Naunyn Schmiedebergs Arch Pharmacol 1975;289(2):149–56.
39. Ginj M, Zhang H, Waser B, et al. Radiolabeled somatostatin receptor antagonists are preferable to agonists for in vivo peptide receptor targeting of tumors. Proc Natl Acad Sci U S A 2006;103(44):16436–41.
40. Mansi R, Wang X, Forrer F, et al. Evaluation of a 1,4,7,10-tetraazacyclododecane-1,4,7,10-tetraacetic acid-conjugated bombesin-based radioantagonist for the labeling with single-photon emission computed tomography, positron emission

tomography, and therapeutic radionuclides. Clin Cancer Res 2009;15(16):5240–9.

41. Millar JB, Rozengurt E. Chronic desensitization to bombesin by progressive down-regulation of bombesin receptors in Swiss 3T3 cells. Distinction from acute desensitization. J Biol Chem 1990;265(20): 12052–8.

42. Kahkonen E, Jambor I, Kemppainen J, et al. In vivo imaging of prostate cancer using [68Ga]-labeled bombesin analog BAY86-7548. Clin Cancer Res 2013;19(19):5434–43.

43. Ambrosini V, Fani M, Fanti S, et al. Radiopeptide imaging and therapy in Europe. J Nucl Med 2011; 52(Suppl 2):42S–55S.

44. Mansi R, Wang X, Forrer F, et al. Development of a potent DOTA-conjugated bombesin antagonist for targeting GRPr-positive tumours. Eur J Nucl Med Mol Imaging 2011;38(1):97–107.

45. Baratto L, Duan H, Laudicella R, et al. Physiological (68)Ga-RM2 uptake in patients with biochemically recurrent prostate cancer: an atlas of semi-quantitative measurements. Eur J Nucl Med Mol Imaging 2020;47(1):115–22.

46. Roivainen A, Kahkonen E, Luoto P, et al. Plasma pharmacokinetics, whole-body distribution, metabolism, and radiation dosimetry of 68Ga bombesin antagonist BAY 86-7548 in healthy men. J Nucl Med 2013;54(6):867–72.

47. Gnesin S, Cicone F, Mitsakis P, et al. First in-human radiation dosimetry of the gastrin-releasing peptide (GRP) receptor antagonist (68)Ga-NODAGA-MJ9. EJNMMI Res 2018;8(1):108.

48. Lantry LE, Cappelletti E, Maddalena ME, et al. 177Lu-AMBA: synthesis and characterization of a selective 177Lu-labeled GRP-R agonist for systemic radiotherapy of prostate cancer. J Nucl Med 2006; 47(7):1144–52.

49. Maecke HR, Hofmann M, Haberkorn U. (68)Ga-labeled peptides in tumor imaging. J Nucl Med 2005;46(Suppl 1):172S-8S.

50. Reubi JC, Macke HR, Krenning EP. Candidates for peptide receptor radiotherapy today and in the future. J Nucl Med 2005;46(Suppl 1):67S–75S.

51. Heppeler A, Froidevaux S, Eberle AN, et al. Receptor targeting for tumor localisation and therapy with radiopeptides. Curr Med Chem 2000;7(9): 971–94.

52. Force USPST, Grossman DC, Curry SJ, et al. Screening for prostate cancer: US preventive services task force recommendation statement. JAMA 2018;319(18):1901–13.

53. Bekelman JE, Rumble RB, Chen RC, et al. Clinically localized prostate cancer: ASCO clinical practice guideline endorsement of an american urological association/american society for radiation oncology/society of urologic oncology guideline. J Clin Oncol 2018;36(32):3251–8.

54. Trabulsi EJ, Rumble RB, Jadvar H, et al. Optimum imaging strategies for advanced prostate cancer: ASCO guideline. J Clin Oncol 2020;38(17):1963–96.

55. Touijer KA, Michaud L, Alvarez HAV, et al. Prospective study of the radiolabeled GRPR antagonist BAY86-7548 for positron emission tomography/computed tomography imaging of newly diagnosed prostate cancer. Eur Urol Oncol 2019;2(2):166–73.

56. Fassbender TF, Schiller F, Zamboglou C, et al. Voxel-based comparison of [(68)Ga]Ga-RM2-PET/CT and [(68)Ga]Ga-PSMA-11-PET/CT with histopathology for diagnosis of primary prostate cancer. EJNMMI Res 2020;10(1):62.

57. Mapelli P, Ghezzo S, Samanes Gajate AM, et al. 68)Ga-PSMA and (68)Ga-DOTA-RM2 PET/MRI in recurrent prostate cancer: diagnostic performance and association with clinical and histopathological data. Cancers (Basel) 2022;14(2). https://doi.org/10.3390/cancers14020334.

58. Baratto L, Duan H, Hatami N, et al. 68Ga-RM2 PET/CT in patients with newly diagnosed intermediate- or high-risk prostate cancer. J Nucl Med 2020; 61(Supplement 1):1261.

59. Cookson MS, Aus G, Burnett AL, et al. Variation in the definition of biochemical recurrence in patients treated for localized prostate cancer: the american urological association prostate guidelines for localized prostate cancer update panel report and recommendations for a standard in the reporting of surgical outcomes. J Urol 2007;177(2):540–5.

60. Roach M 3rd, Hanks G, Thames H Jr, et al. Defining biochemical failure following radiotherapy with or without hormonal therapy in men with clinically localized prostate cancer: recommendations of the RTOG-ASTRO phoenix consensus conference. Int J Radiat Oncol Biol Phys 2006;65(4):965–74.

61. Caire AA, Sun L, Ode O, et al. Delayed prostate-specific antigen recurrence after radical prostatectomy: how to identify and what are their clinical outcomes? Urology 2009;74(3):643–7.

62. Crocerossa F, Marchioni M, Novara G, et al. Detection rate of prostate specific membrane antigen tracers for positron emission tomography/computerized tomography in prostate cancer biochemical recurrence: a systematic review and network meta-analysis. J Urol 2021;205(2):356–69.

63. Baratto L, Song H, Duan H, et al. PSMA- and GRPR-targeted PET: results from 50 patients with biochemically recurrent prostate cancer. J Nucl Med 2021. https://doi.org/10.2967/jnumed.120.259630.

64. Wieser G, Popp I, Christian Rischke H, et al. Diagnosis of recurrent prostate cancer with PET/CT imaging using the gastrin-releasing peptide receptor antagonist (68)Ga-RM2: preliminary results in patients with negative or inconclusive [(18)F]Fluoroethylcholine-PET/CT. Eur J Nucl Med Mol Imaging 2017;44(9):1463–72.

65. Maina T, Bergsma H, Kulkarni HR, et al. Preclinical and first clinical experience with the gastrin-releasing peptide receptor-antagonist [(6)(8)Ga] SB3 and PET/CT. Eur J Nucl Med Mol Imaging 2016;43(5):964–73.

66. Meller B, Bremmer F, Sahlmann CO, et al. Alterations in androgen deprivation enhanced prostate-specific membrane antigen (PSMA) expression in prostate cancer cells as a target for diagnostics and therapy. EJNMMI Res 2015;5(1):66.

67. Nock BA, Kaloudi A, Lymperis E, et al. Theranostic perspectives in prostate cancer with the gastrin-releasing peptide receptor antagonist NeoBOMB1: preclinical and first clinical results. J Nucl Med 2017;58(1):75–80.

68. Dalm SU, Bakker IL, de Blois E, et al. 68Ga/177Lu-NeoBOMB1, a novel radiolabeled GRPR antagonist for theranostic use in oncology. J Nucl Med 2017; 58(2):293–9.

69. Gruber L, Jimenez-Franco LD, Decristoforo C, et al. MITIGATE-NeoBOMB1, a Phase I/IIa study to evaluate safety, Pharmacokinetics, and preliminary imaging of (68)Ga-NeoBOMB1, a gastrin-releasing peptide receptor antagonist, in GIST patients. J Nucl Med 2020;61(12):1749–55.

70. Mitran B, Varasteh Z, Abouzayed A, et al. Bispecific GRPR-antagonistic anti-PSMA/GRPR heterodimer for PET and SPECT diagnostic imaging of prostate cancer. Cancers (Basel) 2019;11(9). https://doi.org/10.3390/cancers11091371.

71. Lundmark F, Abouzayed A, Mitran B, et al. Heterodimeric radiotracer targeting PSMA and GRPR for imaging of prostate cancer-optimization of the affinity towards PSMA by linker modification in murine model. Pharmaceutics 2020;12(7). https://doi.org/10.3390/pharmaceutics12070614.

72. Ye S, Li H, Hu K, et al. Radiosynthesis and biological evaluation of 18F-labeled bispecific heterodimer targeted dual gastrin-releasing peptide receptor and prostate-specific membrane antigen for prostate cancer imaging. Nucl Med Commun 2022;43(3): 323–31.

73. Abouzayed A, Yim CB, Mitran B, et al. Synthesis and preclinical evaluation of radio-iodinated GRPR/PSMA bispecific heterodimers for the theranostics application in prostate cancer. Pharmaceutics 2019;11(7). https://doi.org/10.3390/pharmaceutics11070358.

Feasibility of Global Assessment of Bone Metastases in Prostate Cancer with ^{18}F-Sodium Fluoride-PET/Computed Tomography

Benjamin Koa, MD[a,1], William Y. Raynor, MD[a,b,1], Peter Sang Uk Park, BA[a,c],
Austin J. Borja, BA[a,c], Sachi Singhal, MD[a,d], Angie Kuang, BS[a],
Vincent Zhang, BA[a], Thomas J. Werner, MSE[a],
Abass Alavi, MD, MD (Hon), PhD (Hon), DSc (Hon)[a],
Mona-Elisabeth Revheim, MD, PhD, MHA[a,e,f],*

KEYWORDS

- Prostate cancer • Bone metastasis • NaF • PET/CT • ALP • PSA

KEY POINTS

- Global disease assessment facilitates an objective evaluation of overall disease activity at the time of diagnosis and at follow up, providing a more straightforward approach to determine response to therapy compared to a lesion-based analysis.
- Dedicated software is available that can not only provide a rapid, semi-automatic method of segmenting PET-avid lesions but can also perform partial volume correction, which is necessary to overcome the partial volume effect, which causes underestimation of uptake in small lesions.
- ^{18}F-sodium fluoride (NaF)-PET/CT is more sensitive than conventional bone scintigraphy for identification of skeletal metastases caused by prostate cancer. However, direct imaging of tumor cells with prostate-specific membrane antigen (PSMA) tracers is expected to surpass either method for the purpose of prostate cancer staging.

INTRODUCTION

Prostate cancer (PCa) is the second most common cancer in men.[1] Although disease localized to the prostate has a 5-year survival rate of approximately 100%, metastatic disease has a 5-year survival rate of 29.3%.[2] The presence of cancer cells in the red marrow leads to osteoblastic reaction and therefore increased new bone formation.[3] Knowledge of plain radiography can be used to detect bone metastases; early skeletal lesions are difficult or impossible to visualize.[4] Planar imaging and single-photon emission tomography (SPECT) with ^{99m}Tc-methylene diphosphonate (^{99m}Tc-MDP) (or other conventional bone tracers) have commonly been used to

[a] Department of Radiology, Hospital of the University of Pennsylvania, 3400 Spruce Street, Philadelphia, PA 19104, USA; [b] Department of Radiology, Rutgers Robert Wood Johnson Medical School, 1 Robert Wood Johnson Place, MEB #404, New Brunswick, NJ 08901, USA; [c] Perelman School of Medicine at the University of Pennsylvania, 3400 Civic Center Boulevard, Philadelphia, PA 19104, USA; [d] Department of Medicine, Crozer-Chester Medical Center, 1 Medical Center Boulevard, Upland, PA 19013, USA; [e] Division of Radiology and Nuclear Medicine, Oslo University Hospital, Sognsvannsveien 20, Oslo 0372, Norway; [f] Institute for Clinical Medicine, University of Oslo, Postbox 4950, Nydalen, Oslo 0424, Norway
[1] These authors contributed equally to this work.
* Corresponding author. Institute for Clinical Medicine, University of Oslo, Postbox 4950, Nydalen, Oslo 0424, Norway
E-mail address: mona.elisabeth.revheim@ous-hf.no

PET Clin 17 (2022) 631–640
https://doi.org/10.1016/j.cpet.2022.07.007
1556-8598/22/

detect areas of increased bone formation associated with metastasis due to their high sensitivity compared with radiography.[5] However, the low specificity of this technique has necessitated corroboration with other imaging modalities, such as computed tomography (CT) and MRI.[6]

PET with ^{18}F-sodium fluoride (NaF), a bone-seeking radiopharmaceutical, has many advantages over ^{99m}Tc-MDP SPECT.[7–9] NaF is exchanged with the hydroxyl (OH⁻) group of hydroxyapatite and then adsorbed to the early phase of the microcalcification process.[10] NaF-PET/CT provides images with superior spatial and contrast resolution, resulting in higher sensitivity and specificity compared with ^{99m}Tc-MDP scintigraphy.[6,10] In addition, faster skeletal uptake of NaF by bone allows early imaging by PET.[6] Furthermore, PET provides images that can be quantified by generating, eg, standardized uptake values (SUVs).[5] These advantages have led to a growing interest in NaF-PET/CT for assessing skeletal disorders and diseases. Detection of metastases is important in PCa as it impacts clinical management. The utility of PET/CT in metastatic PCa was shown in a US registry study on metastatic PCa as NaF PET/CT had not only replaced the use of other advanced imaging techniques in 50% of cases but also had led to treatment plan modifications in 76% of those cases.[11] In addition, NaF PET/CT was shown to be a predictive marker for overall survival and occurrence of bone-related events during chemotherapy.[12] Global assessment, which has been applied in a variety of other domains, is a method of quantifying total disease activity using metabolic and volumetric parameters.[13] However, no studies have been performed correlating global disease assessment of skeletal metastases in PCa to clinical biomarkers, such as alkaline phosphatase (ALP) and prostate-specific antigen (PSA).

In this study, we aimed to determine the feasibility of performing a semiautomatic method of quantification for the global assessment of skeletal metastases in patients with PCa. Specifically, we evaluate the association of PET parameters with established markers of metastatic bone disease in PCa, ALP, and PSA.

METHODS
Study Setting

We examined NaF-PET/CT scans of 32 patients with PCa who were referred to the Department of Radiology for suspected skeletal metastasis. A total of 45 patients were referred, of which 32 were included in this study as they had undergone full-body imaging, whereas the other 13 were excluded as they had only undergone upper body imaging. Approval was obtained from the University of Pennsylvania Institutional Review Board, and all work was performed in compliance with the Health Insurance Portability and Accountability Act (HIPAA).

Image Acquisition

Imaging of all patients was performed on integrated PET/CT scanners at the Hospital of the University of Pennsylvania (Gemini TF; Philips Healthcare, Best, The Netherlands). Approximately 60 min after intravenous administration of 3.0 MBq/kg of tracer, whole-body images were acquired to include the whole skeleton. Along with PET, an unenhanced low-dose CT was performed for the purposes of PET attenuation correction and assessment of structural findings.

Image and Statistical Analysis

Researchers who were blinded to clinical information performed segmentation of NaF-avid skeletal metastases using a semiautomatic approach. An iterative adaptive thresholding algorithm was used to delineate lesions identified by the researchers (ROVER software; ABX GmbH, Radeberg, Germany) (**Figs. 1** and **2**). Subvolumes were manually defined to encompass NaF-avid lesions suspicious for metastasis while avoiding areas of tracer accumulation secondary to degenerative joint disease, vascular calcification, urinary excretion, and other benign causes. The initial threshold was set at 40% of the maximum standardized uptake value (SUVmax) within each subvolume. A detailed explanation of how this initial threshold was iteratively modified to achieve an optimal threshold delineating focal uptake from background uptake is described by Hofheinz and colleagues.[14] Correction for the partial volume effect was carried out automatically based on background uptake and spill-out activity. Based on data generated by this software, PET parameters including the metabolically active volume (MAV), SUVmax, mean metabolic volume product (MVPmean = SUVmean × MAV), and partial volume-corrected MVPmean (cMVPmean = cSUV mean × MAV) were calculated. Global parameters reflecting total disease activity were defined as the sum of each parameter across all lesions within the structures assessed. Using Stata/MP Version 16 (StataCorp), Pearson correlations were used to assess associations between global NaF-PET parameters and the laboratory values, ALP and PSA.

RESULTS

The patient population examined included 32 men with ages ranging from 55 to 82 years (mean 69.3,

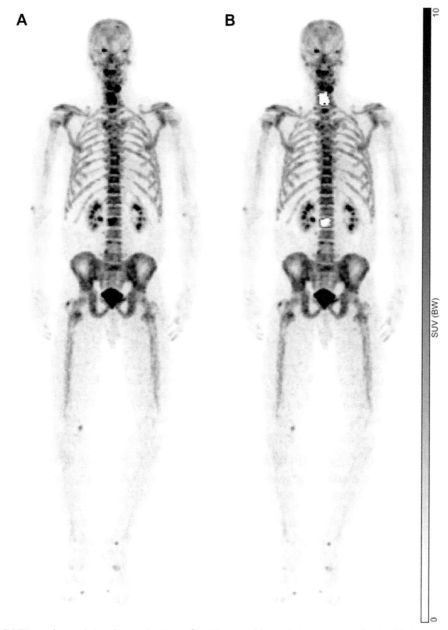

Fig. 1. NaF-PET maximum intensity projection of a 60-year-old prostate cancer patient with bone metastases before (*A*) and after (*B*) segmentation with ROVER software. Global cMVPmean was found to be 231, ALP was 61 U/L, and PSA was 0.4 ng/mL. *Abbreviation:* SUV (BW), standardized uptake value (body weight).

standard deviation [SD] 6.7). Correlations between PET parameters and ALP and PSA are shown in **Table 1**. According to Pearson correlational analysis, ALP was significantly and positively correlated with global MVPmean ($r = 0.49$, $p = 0.004$, **Fig. 3**), cMVPmean ($r = 0.48$, $p = 0.005$, **Fig. 4**), and MAV ($r = 0.38$, $p = 0.03$, **Fig. 5**). However, PSA was not correlated to these PET metrics ($r = 0.23$, $p = 0.22$; $r = 0.25$, $p = 0.17$; $r = 0.10$, $p = 0.60$, respectively, **Figs. 6–8**). In addition, no

significant correlation was observed between SUV-max and cSUVmax and either ALP ($r = 0.21$, $p = 0.26$; $r = 0.10$, $p = 0.58$, respectively) or PSA ($r = 0.21$, $p = 0.24$; $r = 0.18$, $p = 0.33$, respectively).

DISCUSSION

In this study, we investigated the feasibility of a semiautomatic method of a global quantification of bone metastases in patients with PCa and the

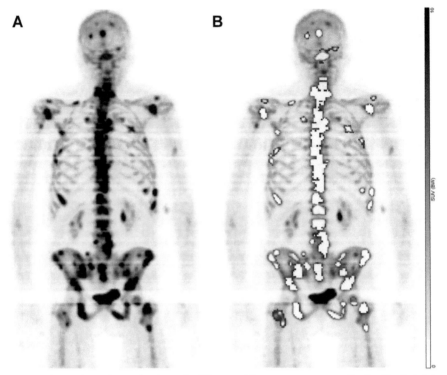

Fig. 2. NaF-PET maximum intensity projection of a 72-year-old prostate cancer patient with skeletal metastases before (*A*) and after (*B*) segmentation with ROVER software. Global cMVPmean was found to be 2073, ALP was 148 U/L, and PSA was 16.9 ng/mL. *Abbreviation:* SUV (BW), standardized uptake value (body weight).

association between global NaF-PET parameters and established blood markers of metastatic bone disease in PCa. There was a statistically significant positive correlation between global MVPmean, cMVPmean, and MAV measurements

Table 1
Pearson correlation analysis

PET Parameter	Pearson *r*	*p*-value
MVPmean vs ALP	0.49	0.004
cMVPmean vs ALP	0.48	0.005
MAV vs ALP	0.38	0.03
SUVmax vs ALP	0.21	0.26
cSUVmax vs ALP	0.10	0.58
MVPmean vs PSA	0.23	0.22
cMVPmean vs PSA	0.25	0.17
MAV vs PSA	0.10	0.60
SUVmax vs PSA	0.21	0.24
cSUVmax vs PSA	0.18	0.33

This table shows Pearson *r* and *p*-values for parameters generated from this research project.

and ALP levels, indicating the validity of this approach.

To the best of our knowledge, few studies have investigated the relationship between NaF-PET parameters and markers of metastatic bone disease. In one study on the repeatability of NaF-PET/CT parameters and biochemical bone markers, the authors found that SUVmean, SUVmax, and whole body NaF skeletal tumor burden did not correlate with any of the biochemical tumor or bone remodeling markers.[15] However, the main concern about these findings is that conventional methods of PET quantification are adversely impacted by the limited spatial resolution of PET which leads to underestimating the true tumor burden and inaccurate results.[16,17] SUVmax measurements are based on the highest metabolic activity of a single voxel within a region of interest and thus may not accurately represent the overall uptake in the lesion of interest.[18] With our analysis scheme, we found a relatively strong correlation between NaF parameters and ALP using MVPmean, cMVPmean, and MAV but not for SUVmax. By conducting this research, we have introduced a new approach for assessing the global disease burden and quantifying the metabolic

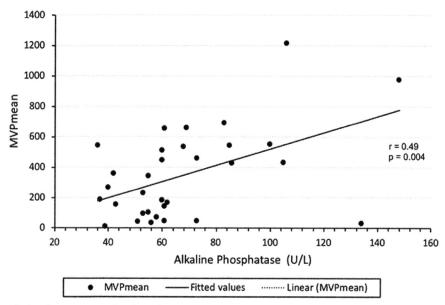

Fig. 3. Correlation between ALP levels and MVPmean as measured on NaF-PET images with ROVER software.

activity of skeletal metastases in PCa. Global PET quantitative methods using partial volume-corrected values with metabolic and volumetric parameters have been shown to provide more accurate measures of systemic disease burden.[16,17] Our study is the first to show the potential of global NaF parameters in the evaluation of metastatic PCa. Studies on skeletal metastasis in other cancers have reported global uptake values that are consistent with our study.[19–23] Therefore, additional studies are warranted to corroborate and

further validate this novel approach in metastatic PCa.

The relationship between NaF-PET parameters and metastatic bone disease markers in PCa has been investigated in the treatment response of castrate-resistant neoplasms.[24,25] These studies have shown a correlation between the changes in mean SUVmax and ALP; however, there are conflicting data to support the presence of any correlation between mean SUVmax and PSA.[24,25] ALP is a marker of bone turnover and

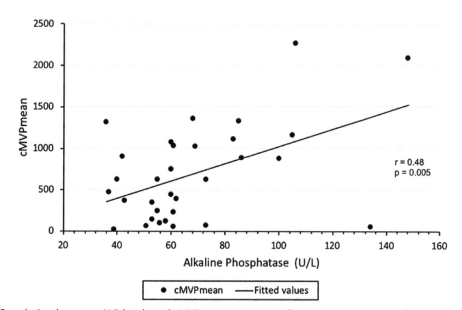

Fig. 4. Correlation between ALP levels and cMVPmean as measured on NaF-PET images with ROVER software.

636 Koa et al

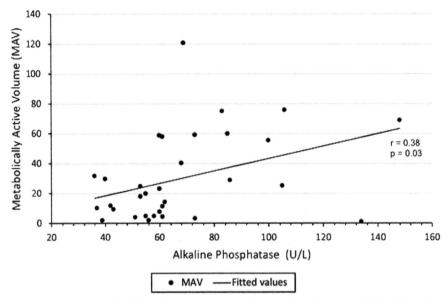

Fig. 5. Correlation between ALP levels and MAV as measured on NaF-PET images with ROVER software.

osteoblastic activity and has been employed as a test that reflects bone metastatic tumor load.[26] Moreover, numerous studies have shown an association of ALP levels to overall survival and disease progression in metastatic castration-resistant PCa.[27–32] As ALP levels correlate with the degree of bone metastatic burden and are elevated in patients with metastasis, we expected a significant correlation between global NaF uptake and such blood markers. Therefore, our findings are very much in line with this speculated hypothesis. PSA is another biomarker commonly used in

metastatic PCa as its levels have also been expected to reflect disease burden and prognosis.[30,33,34] Although our study did not observe any correlation between PET parameters and PSA, an association between positive metastatic NaF uptake and low PSA levels has been previously reported, with NaF-PET/CT revealing potential sites of occult osseous metastases and exhibiting high sensitivity over traditional bone scans.[35] As such, the use of NaF-PET at levels of PSA even lower than 20 ng/ml has been recommended for the detection of bone metastases.[36]

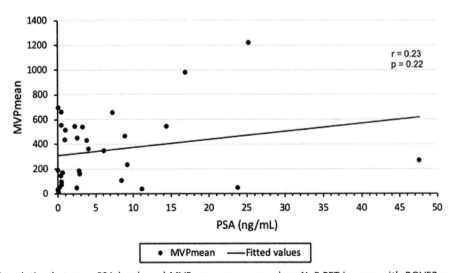

Fig. 6. Correlation between PSA levels and MVPmean as measured on NaF-PET images with ROVER software.

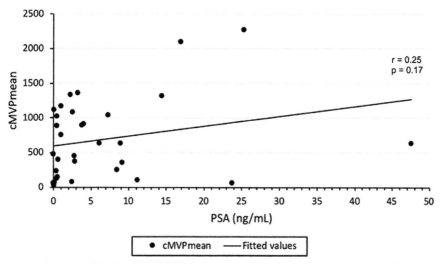

Fig. 7. Correlation between PSA levels and cMVPmean as measured on NaF-PET images with ROVER software.

Additional research on the association among positive NaF-PET findings, PSA levels, and therapeutic response may further reveal the applicability and relationship of NaF-PET with PSA.

Our study is not without limitations. First is the challenge of differentiating metastatic lesions from degenerative lesions in our segmentation method. For instance, NaF uptake in degenerative parts of the body, such as lumbar facet joints has been well reported in the literature.[37,38] However, benign causes of NaF uptake often differ from that of bone metastases in spatial pattern; for example, benign uptakes are common in osteophytes, weight-bearing aspects of the joint, or site of enthesopathy. On the contrary, malignant uptakes are found in axial and appendicular bone with red marrow distribution or posterior aspect of the vertebral body.[39,40] Furthermore,

differentiation between benign and malignant lesions has been studied by setting a quantitatively discriminative threshold.[41,42] As such, the specificity of NaF-PET/CT can be enhanced by the discernment of the operator and quantitative thresholding of the segmentation. Incorporation of artificial intelligence and machine learning to measure tumor burden and distinguish malignant from benign lesions may be an additional promising step toward achieving greater precision in the detection of metastatic lesions.[43,44]

Another limitation was that our study did not examine the clinical data that were generated in this population. However, this retrospective research study was initiated to test and validate a new image analysis scheme for quantifying the extent of metastatic lesions in the skeletal structures. Therefore, the main aim of this

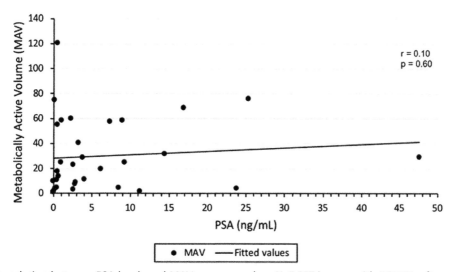

Fig. 8. Correlation between PSA levels and MAV as measured on NaF-PET images with ROVER software.

investigation was technical, and not biological, in nature. As such, we made no effort to examine the clinical data that were generated in this population.

The novel approach using global assessment can also be adapted for more specific PET tracers. Various PET radiotracers have been studied in the evaluation of metastatic PCa such as the depiction of prostate-specific membrane antigen with gallium-68 and fluorine-18, expression of androgen receptors with 16β-18F-fluoro-5α-dihydrotestosterone, and synthetic of fatty acids with ^{11}C-acetate. With the impact the presence and progress of metastasis has on the clinical management of PCa, further studies would be warranted to corroborate this novel approach.

CLINICS CARE POINTS

- Compared to bone scintigraphy with ^{99m}Tc-methylene diphosphonate, NaF-PET/CT demonstrates superior tumor-to-background uptake, greater spatial resolution, and improved methods of quantification.

- SUVmean, which represents an average of the activity within a particular region of interest, is more reliable than SUVmax, which represents the value of the hottest voxel and may not be representative of the overall lesional activity.

- Global assessment, calculated by combining the activity of all pathological lesions, is an efficient and reliable measure of total disease activity and cen be used to assess disease progression and response to treatment.

CONFLICT OF DISCLOSURE

The authors have no conflict of interest to disclose.

REFERENCES

1. Barsouk A, Padala SA, Vakiti A, et al. Epidemiology, staging and management of prostate cancer. Med Sci Basel Switz 2020;8(3). https://doi.org/10.3390/medsci8030028.
2. Damodaran S, Kyriakopoulos CE, Jarrard DF. Newly diagnosed metastatic prostate cancer: has the paradigm changed? Urol Clin North Am 2017;44(4): 611–21.
3. Macedo F, Ladeira K, Pinho F, et al. Bone metastases: an overview. Oncol Rev 2017;11(1). https://doi.org/10.4081/oncol.2017.321.
4. Cook GJ, Goh V. Functional and hybrid imaging of bone metastases. J Bone Miner Res 2018;33(6): 961–72. https://doi.org/10.1002/jbmr.3444.
5. Langsteger W, Rezaee A, Pirich C, et al. 18F-NaF-PET/CT and 99mTc-MDP bone scintigraphy in the detection of bone metastases in prostate cancer. Semin Nucl Med 2016;46(6):491–501.
6. Bastawrous S, Bhargava P, Behnia F, et al. Newer PET application with an old tracer: role of 18F-NaF skeletal PET/CT in oncologic practice. RadioGraphics 2014;34(5):1295–316.
7. Zhang V, Koa B, Borja AJ, et al. Diagnosis and monitoring of osteoporosis with total-body 18F-sodium fluoride-PET/CT. PET Clin 2020;15(4):487–96.
8. Raynor WY, Borja AJ, Rojulpote C, et al. 18F-sodium fluoride: an emerging tracer to assess active vascular microcalcification. J Nucl Cardiol 2020. https://doi.org/10.1007/s12350-020-02138-9.
9. Mayer M, Borja AJ, Hancin EC, et al. Imaging atherosclerosis by PET, with emphasis on the role of FDG and NaF as potential biomarkers for this disorder. Front Physiol 2020;11. https://doi.org/10.3389/fphys.2020.511391.
10. Farolfi A, Hadaschik B, Hamdy FC, et al. Positron emission tomography and whole-body magnetic resonance imaging for metastasis-directed therapy in hormone-sensitive oligometastatic prostate cancer after primary radical treatment: a systematic review. Eur Urol Oncol 2021;4(5):714–30.
11. Hillner BE, Siegel BA, Hanna L, et al. 18F-fluoride PET used for treatment monitoring of systemic cancer therapy: results from the National Oncologic PET Registry. J Nucl Med 2015;56(2):222–8.
12. Etchebehere EC, Araujo JC, Fox PS, et al. Prognostic factors in patients treated with 223Ra: the role of skeletal tumor burden on baseline 18F-fluoride PET/CT in predicting overall survival. J Nucl Med 2015;56(8):1177–84. https://doi.org/10.2967/jnumed.115.158626.
13. Høilund-Carlsen PF, Edenbrandt L, Alavi A. Global disease score (GDS) is the name of the game. Eur J Nucl Med Mol Imaging 2019;46(9):1768–72. https://doi.org/10.1007/s00259-019-04383-8.
14. Hofheinz F, Pötzsch C, Oehme L, et al. Automatic volume delineation in oncological PET. evaluation of a dedicated software tool and comparison with manual delineation in clinical data sets. Nukl Nucl Med 2012;51(1):9–16. https://doi.org/10.3413/Nukmed-0419-11-07.
15. Wassberg C, Lubberink M, Sörensen J, et al. Repeatability of quantitative parameters of 18F-fluoride PET/CT and biochemical tumour and specific bone remodelling markers in prostate cancer bone metastases. EJNMMI Res 2017;7. https://doi.org/10.1186/s13550-017-0289-9.
16. Hofheinz F, Langner J, Petr J, et al. A method for model-free partial volume correction in oncological

PET. EJNMMI Res 2012;2(1):16. https://doi.org/10.1186/2191-219X-2-16.

17. Torigian DA, Lopez RF, Alapati S, et al. Feasibility and performance of novel software to quantify metabolically active volumes and 3D partial volume corrected SUV and metabolic volumetric products of spinal bone marrow metastases on 18F-FDG-PET/CT. Hell J Nucl Med 2011;14(1):8–14.

18. Vanderhoek M, Perlman SB, Jeraj R. Impact of the definition of peak standardized uptake value on quantification of treatment response. J Nucl Med 2012;53(1):4–11. https://doi.org/10.2967/jnumed.111.093443.

19. Letellier A, Johnson AC, Kit NH, et al. Uptake of radium-223 dichloride and early [18F]NaF PET response are driven by baseline [18F]NaF parameters: a pilot study in castration-resistant prostate cancer patients. Mol Imaging Biol 2018;20(3):482–91.

20. Zirakchian Zadeh M, Østergaard B, Raynor WY, et al. Comparison of 18F-sodium fluoride uptake in the whole bone, pelvis, and femoral neck of multiple myeloma patients before and after high-dose therapy and conventional-dose chemotherapy. Eur J Nucl Med Mol Imaging 2020;47(12):2846–55. https://doi.org/10.1007/s00259-020-04768-0.

21. Brito AE, Santos A, Sasse AD, et al. 18 F-Fluoride PET/CT tumor burden quantification predicts survival in breast cancer. Oncotarget 2017;8(22):36001–11.

22. Zadeh MZ, Raynor WY, Seraj SM, et al. Evolving roles of fluorodeoxyglucose and sodium fluoride in assessment of multiple myeloma patients: introducing a novel method of pet quantification to overcome shortcomings of the existing approaches. PET Clin 2019;14(3):341–52.

23. Zadeh MZ, Seraj SM, Østergaard B, et al. Prognostic significance of 18F-sodium fluoride in newly diagnosed multiple myeloma patients. Am J Nucl Med Mol Imaging 2020;10(4):151–60.

24. Yu EY, Duan F, Muzi M, et al. Castration-resistant prostate cancer bone metastasis response measured by 18F-fluoride PET after treatment with dasatinib and correlation with progression-free survival: results from American College of Radiology Imaging Network 6687. J Nucl Med 2015;56(3):354–60.

25. Cook GJ, Parker C, Chua S, et al. 18F-fluoride PET: changes in uptake as a method to assess response in bone metastases from castrate-resistant prostate cancer patients treated with 223Ra-chloride (Alpharadin). EJNMMI Res 2011;1:4. https://doi.org/10.1186/2191-219X-1-4.

26. Mori K, Janisch F, Parizi MK, et al. Prognostic value of alkaline phosphatase in hormone-sensitive prostate cancer: a systematic review and meta-analysis. Int J Clin Oncol 2020;25(2):247–57.

27. Fizazi K, Massard C, Smith M, et al. Bone-related parameters are the main prognostic factors for overall survival in men with bone metastases from castration-resistant prostate cancer. Eur Urol 2015;68(1):42–50.

28. Chi KN, Kheoh T, Ryan CJ, et al. A prognostic index model for predicting overall survival in patients with metastatic castration-resistant prostate cancer treated with abiraterone acetate after docetaxel. Ann Oncol 2016;27(3):454–60.

29. Guinney J, Wang T, Laajala TD, et al. Prediction of overall survival for patients with metastatic castration-resistant prostate cancer: development of a prognostic model through a crowdsourced challenge with open clinical trial data. Lancet Oncol 2017;18(1):132–42.

30. Halabi S, Lin CY, Kelly WK, et al. Updated prognostic model for predicting overall survival in first-line chemotherapy for patients with metastatic castration-resistant prostate cancer. J Clin Oncol 2014;32(7):671–7.

31. D'Oronzo S, Brown J, Coleman R. The value of biomarkers in bone metastasis. Eur J Cancer Care (Engl) 2017;26(6). https://doi.org/10.1111/ecc.12725.

32. Li D, Lv H, Hao X, et al. Prognostic value of serum alkaline phosphatase in the survival of prostate cancer: evidence from a meta-analysis. Cancer Manag Res 2018;10:3125–39.

33. Koo KC, Park SU, Kim KH, et al. Predictors of survival in prostate cancer patients with bone metastasis and extremely high prostate-specific antigen levels. Prostate Int 2015;3(1):10–5.

34. Lojanapiwat B, Anutrakulchai W, Chongruksut W, et al. Correlation and diagnostic performance of the prostate-specific antigen level with the diagnosis, aggressiveness, and bone metastasis of prostate cancer in clinical practice. Prostate Int 2014;2(3):133–9.

35. Jadvar H, Desai B, Ji L, et al. Prospective evaluation of 18F-NaF and 18F-FDG PET/CT in detection of occult metastatic disease in biochemical recurrence of prostate cancer. Clin Nucl Med 2012;37(7):637–43.

36. Sarikaya I, Sarikaya A, Elgazzar AH, et al. Prostate-specific antigen cutoff value for ordering sodium fluoride positron emission tomography/computed tomography bone scan in patients with prostate cancer. World J Nucl Med 2018;17(4):281–5.

37. Mabray MC, Brus-Ramer M, Behr SC, et al. (18)F-Sodium fluoride PET-CT hybrid imaging of the lumbar facet joints: tracer uptake and degree of correlation to CT-graded arthropathy. World J Nucl Med 2016;15(2):85–90.

38. Spirig JM, Hüllner M, Cornaz F, et al. 18F-Fluoride PET/MR for painful lumbar facet joint degeneration

- a randomized controlled clinical trial. Spine J 2021. https://doi.org/10.1016/j.spinee.2021.11.014.

39. Wolff JM, Zimny M, Borchers H, et al. Is prostate-specific antigen a reliable marker of bone metastasis in patients with newly diagnosed cancer of the prostate? Eur Urol 1998;33(4):376–81.

40. Panagiotidis E, Lam K, Mistry A, et al. Skeletal metastases and benign mimics on NaF PET/CT: a pictorial review. AJR Am J Roentgenol 2018;211(1): W64–74. https://doi.org/10.2214/AJR.17.19110.

41. Lin C, Bradshaw T, Perk T, et al. Repeatability of quantitative 18F-NaF PET: a multicenter study. J Nucl Med 2016;57(12):1872–9.

42. Muzahir S, Jeraj R, Liu G, et al. Differentiation of metastatic vs degenerative joint disease using semi-quantitative analysis with (18)F-NaF PET/CT in castrate resistant prostate cancer patients. Am J Nucl Med Mol Imaging 2015;5(2):162–8.

43. Perk T, Bradshaw T, Chen S, et al. Automated classification of benign and malignant lesions in 18F-NaF PET/CT images using machine learning. Phys Med Biol 2018;63(22):225019.

44. Polymeri E, Kjölhede H, Enqvist O, et al. Artificial intelligence-based measurements of PET/CT imaging biomarkers are associated with disease-specific survival of high-risk prostate cancer patients. Scand J Urol 2021;55(6):427–33.

Dual-Tracer PET-Computed Tomography Imaging for Precision Radio-Molecular Theranostics of Prostate Cancer
A Futuristic Perspective

Aadil Adnan, MD[a,b], Sandip Basu, DNB[a,b],*

KEYWORDS

- Prostate carcinoma • Dual-tracer PET-CT • Radio-molecular theranostics
- Metastatic castration-resistant prostate carcinoma (mCRPC) • ^{68}Ga-PSMA-11 • FDG PET-CT
- ^{177}Lu-PSMA • Peptide receptor radioligand therapy (PRLT)

KEY POINTS

- Conventional imaging in prostate carcinoma includes multiparametric magnetic resonance imaging (mpMRI), computed tomography (CT), and transrectal ultrasonography (TRUS). mpMRI specifically with endorectal coil is quite sensitive for detecting primary intraprostatic lesion and local invasion to seminal vesicles, pelvic wall, and other pelvic viscera. .
- PET imaging has opened new avenues in prostate carcinoma in detecting: primary lesion, early biochemical recurrence, metastatic tumor burden, and in devising personalized management.
- Furthermore, noninvasive diagnostic modality is need of the hour for staging and restaging prostate carcinoma as TRUS-guided biopsy sometimes may have life-threatening complications. Importantly, findings on noninvasive investigations could potentially guide selection of biopsy sites.
- Prostate-specific membrane antigen (PSMA) PET/CT in this context has great potential as a "rule out" test for prostate carcinoma in baseline staging while being very useful in restaging and metastatic workup. On the contrary, FDG-PET/CT has prognostic implications particularly in patients with relatively aggressive disease.
- Dual-tracer" PET-CT in prostate cancer (especially in the metastatic setting and metastatic castration-resistant prostate carcinoma) has been used to obtain valuable insights pertaining to tumor biology akin to that in metastatic/advanced neuroendocrine neoplasms, using various tracers in combination with FDG which can potentially help in determining effective treatment modalities to be introduced at appropriate stages in disease course, thereby tailoring precise and personalized approach to disease management.
- Recently a six-tier scoring system incorporating the findings of both PSMA and FDG PET-CT scans was published (the "Pro-PET" Scoring system). The proposed "Pro-PET" score employs a categorical scale comprising of scores 0 to 5 with potential prognostic implications and can guide the practice of precision oncology with its ability to explore overall tumor biology and differentiation status of the disease including dynamic disease prognostication.

a Radiation Medicine Centre (B.A.R.C.), Tata Memorial Hospital Annexe, Jerbai Wadia Road, Parel, Mumbai 400012, India; b Homi Bhabha National Institute, Mumbai, India
* Corresponding author.
E-mail address: drsanb@yahoo.com

PET Clin 17 (2022) 641–652
https://doi.org/10.1016/j.cpet.2022.07.008
1556-8598/22/

INTRODUCTION

Prostate cancer is the second most common malignancy and fifth most common cause of death in men worldwide and the lifetime risk of acquiring prostate cancer in developed countries is approximately one in six men.[1,2] Prostate-specific antigen (PSA) screening has enabled early detection of prostate carcinoma and most patients present with locoregional involvement (~93%) and metastatic disease at diagnosis is present in approximately 4%.[3] Approach toward most of the patients diagnosed with prostate cancer is with curative intent either with radical prostatectomy (RP) or radical radiotherapy (RT) to prostate bed followed by androgen deprivation therapy (ADT). Majority of the patients treated with curative intent have good and lasting disease control; however, many will eventually present with biochemical recurrence (BCR) and metastatic disease.[4] Among patients with BCR and metastatic disease, a substantial proportion in immediate or remote course of disease will develop potentially lethal castration resistant state characterized by biochemical and/ or structural disease progression despite castrate levels of androgen, which is attributed to multifactorial mechanisms including mutation, overexpression and ligand independent activation.[5,6] Risk of recurrent metastatic disease post-curative treatment is substantial in "high risk" patients (characterized by high Gleason score and group, high serum PSA [>20 ng/mL], and metastatic disease at diagnosis).[7–9]

Although much has not changed in the treatment of locoregional and non-metastatic/ metastatic hormone-sensitive prostate carcinoma (HSPC), the present decade has witnessed significant advancement in diagnosis and treatment of metastatic castration-resistant prostate carcinoma (mCRPC) with multiple diagnostic and therapeutic alternatives.[8,10–12] In mCRPC, many classes of medical treatment have proven survival benefit and encompasses: (a) second-generation androgen receptor signaling inhibitors (ARSi)— abiraterone and enzalutamide; (b) chemotherapy with docetaxel and cabazitaxel; and (c) prostate-specific membrane antigen targeting radioligand therapy (PSMA PRLT).[13–18] Hence, it is of critical importance to diagnose recurrent HSPC or mCRPC and its biology, so as to introduce appropriate therapeutic agent early in the disease course to ensure maximum response.

Functional imaging with PET/computed tomography (CT) can detect molecular changes before morphologic changes become apparent on conventional anatomic imaging such as CT or MRI.[19] "Dual/Multi-tracer" PET-CT has been an interesting and intriguing concept and is promising in noninvasive and overall characterization of tumor biology and heterogeneity and has scientifically augmented the practice of precision oncology.[20–22] In prostate carcinoma, particularly in mCRPC setting, dual-tracer PET-CT is useful in selecting patients for chemotherapy, ADT or PSMA PRLT either as monotherapy or as combination therapy, ascertaining differentiation status, staging/restaging, prognostication, and predicting progression/response.

In consonance with the above-mentioned concept, Adnan and Basu have proposed a six-tier scoring system "Pro-PET score" incorporating and integrating the findings of both PSMA and FDG PET-CT scans into scores ranging from 0 to 5.[23] The proposed "Pro-PET" score employs a categorical scale comprising of scores 0 to 5, which is largely based on uptake characteristics of the lesion under question with respect to the recognized reference lesion, where score 1 corresponds to purely PSMA avid disease without FDG uptake in any of the lesions and score 5 indicates purely FDG avid disease without gallium-68 (^{68}Ga)-PSMA uptake in any of the lesions; score 0 indicates normal scan on both ^{68}Ga-PSMA and FDG (**Figs. 1** and **2**). The scoring scheme is further ramified depending upon the disease burden and number of discordant lesions on both ^{68}Ga-PSMA and FDG PET-CT scans (see **Figs. 1** and **2**). The inference thus drawn can be used for stratifying the patients deemed suitable for lutetium-177 (^{177}Lu)-PSMA PRLT as monotherapy or with hormonal adjuvants versus those may or may not be suitable for monotherapy and for the patients falling in right end of the spectrum in whom chemotherapy may be more suitable and PRLT is unlikely to be a single effective therapy as can be comprehended from **Fig. 2**.

The aim of this review was to explore the role of dual-tracer PET-CT, particularly PSMA and FDG (flurodeoxyglucose) in various diagnostic and theranostic aspects and utility of the same for developing a precision oncology model for personalization of various available therapeutic alternatives. Furthermore, we have included few more tracers that were studied in dual-tracer setting. Below is the account of utility of dual-tracer PET-CT for various indications in prostate carcinoma and its impact on clinical management.

Diagnosis

Suspicion of prostate carcinoma is mainly clinical and usually characterized by urinary outflow obstruction leading to increased frequency, urgency, nocturia and incontinence, and in

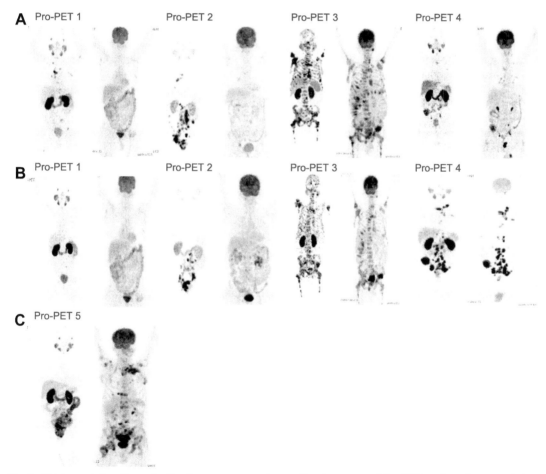

Fig. 1. Spectrum of proposed Pro-PET scoring system by integrating findings of both PSMA and FDG-PET scans in patients with prostate carcinoma. From Adnan A, Basu S. Concept proposal for a six-tier integrated dual-tracer PET-CT (68Ga-PSMA and FDG) image scoring system ("Pro-PET" score) and examining its potential implications in metastatic castration-resistant prostate carcinoma theranostics and prognosis. Nucl Med Commun. 2021 May 1;42(5):566-574.

Fig. 2. Maximum intensity projection images arranged according to proposed Pro-PET scoring scheme and show the responses in each of the subcategories. Row (A) shows baseline 68Ga-PSMA & FDG-PET scans, whereas row (B) shows 68Ga-PSMA and FDG-PET scans post-177Lu-PSMA therapy. Row (C) shows baseline 68Ga-PSMA and FDG-PET scans of patient with Pro-PET score 5 (as the patient was ineligible for 177Lu-PSMA therapy, post-therapy scans were not available). Pro-PET 1 shows complete resolution, Pro-PET 2 shows partial response, Pro-PET 3 shows stable disease, and Pro-PET 4 shows disease progression. From Adnan A, Basu S. Concept proposal for a six-tier integrated dual-tracer PET-CT (68Ga-PSMA and FDG) image scoring system ("Pro-PET" score) and examining its potential implications in metastatic castration-resistant prostate carcinoma theranostics and prognosis. Nucl Med Commun. 2021 May 1;42(5):566-574.

advanced cases may present with hematuria and pathologic fracture particularly in elderly males. PSA with digital rectal examination (DRE) is most widely used modality for screening in such high-risk cases and helps in nearly accurate selection of patients for biopsy, which is gold standard for confirmatory diagnosis. Earlier, DRE was used to guide the tissue sampling in biopsy, but with advancements in imaging, mpMRI and transrectal ultrasound (TRUS) guides biopsy in prostate cancer and significantly betters the diagnostic yield.

Functional imaging has no routine role in initial diagnostic workup of prostate carcinoma. mpMRI is quite sensitive tool for detecting clinically important intraprostatic lesion, which can be targeted for biopsy.[24] However, PSMA PET-CT gives an idea regarding grade of disease preoperatively: in few studies (one retrospective review evaluating PSMA in 72 patients for diagnosis and grading of local prostate cancer and another, a meta-analysis of seven studies comprising 389 patients and assessing diagnostic accuracy of PSMA for initial detection in patients with suspected prostate carcinoma), the predictive accuracy particularly correlated with age of the patient, maximum standardized uptake value (SUVmax) and to a lesser extent with PSA value and maximum dimension of PSMA avid lesion.[25,26] In a still lower proportion of patients, focal high uptake of FDG may indicate malignant lesion and should not be ignored.[27] Kwan and colleagues[25] in their study found the sensitivity of PSMA PET-CT in detecting prostate cancer to be 81.2% that was retrospectively confirmed on RP samples. In a study comprising 6128 men who underwent FDG PET-CT scan for various indications, the incidental FDG uptake in prostate was noted in 1.3%; another meta-analysis and systemic review comprising 47,935 patients reported a pooled prevalence of 1.8% for incidental high FDG uptake in prostate gland and the pooled risk of malignancy with biopsy verification was 62%.[28,29] Hence, it was inferred that incidental high FDG uptake (in one study SUVmax > 6) in prostate should not be ignored and be correlated with serum PSA followed by mpMRI, if clinically indicated thereafter.[30–32] Furthermore, prostatic lesions with higher FDG uptake that turned out to be malignant on biopsy were associated with more aggressive cancer (Gleason score > 7).[33] Hence "dual-tracer" PET-CT using PSMA and FDG can be complementary in initial diagnosis of prostate cancer in both patients suspected for prostate cancer and with incidental high intraprostatic metabolic activity. Other PET tracers targeting cell membrane phospholipids (phosphatidyl choline, carbon C-11 (^{11}C)/fluorine-18 (^{18}F) choline) and amino-acid

transport targeting alanine-serine-cysteine transporter 2 (ASCT2) and L-amino-acid transporter 1 (LAT-1) have no well-defined role in primary diagnosis and is mainly used for BCR and detecting extra-prostatic sites of disease involvement.[34–40] Moreover, choline PET-CT cannot distinguish between benign and malignant lesions.

Staging

mpMRI is a sensitive tool for localizing clinically important lesion for targeted biopsy.[24] mpMRI is the modality of choice for "T-staging" of prostate cancer because it can better show extra-capsular extension, seminal vesicle invasion, and location of lesion in peripheral, transitional, or central zone of prostate. mpMRI, therefore, is the modality of choice for detecting intra-prostatic disease, whereas PET-CT scores better for detecting extra-prostatic and metastatic involvement. It is important to detect extra-prostatic and metastatic disease because at the time of diagnosis: 10% to 20% of patients have locally advanced disease and 8% to 35% patients present with distant metastases, and lymph nodal involvement is reported in approximately 33% of the patients.[41] mpMRI and CT scans which use size criteria and structural morphology for detecting nodal involvement have limited sensitivity with detection rate of less than 40%.[42] Bone scintigraphy with phosphonate-based tracers also has limited sensitivity and specificity mainly because of poor image resolution (which has been to a great alleviated by using ^{18}F-sodium fluoride [NaF] PET-CT) and nonspecific uptake in many metabolic and reactive conditions and is therefore recommended at PSA of 20 ng/mL or more in T1 disease and at PSA 10 ng/mL or more in T2 prostate cancer.[43–45]

Recent studies have shown PSMA PET-CT of having equivalent performance to be complementary to mpMRI in initial staging and hence can be considered in patients in whom MRI is contraindicated.[46] These studies further shown the extent of PSMA uptake to be a function of various risk factors like high Gleason score (>7), high baseline serum PSA levels (>10 ng/mL), and therefore few of the current guidelines recommend PSMA PET-CT before surgery and RT in patients having high-risk features at baseline.[46–49] Furthermore, PSMA PET-CT enabled detection of nodal and bone metastases in 26.7% and 12.2%, respectively.[47] Cumulative evidence indicates that PSMA PET-CT should be a preferred imaging modality for staging patients with intermediate- to high-risk prostate cancer.[50–55] A prospective randomized trial by Hofman and colleagues[51] determined that PSMA PET-CT was 27% (95% confidence interval [CI]: 23–31) more accurate than conventional imaging.

In most of the patients with prostate cancer, PSMA expression is 100 to 1000 times more than normal cells and benign prostatic disorders and increases with increasing tumor stage, grade, and with development of castration resistant state; however, in approximately 5% to 10% of patients PSMA PET-CT is negative and the potential explanation being less than 100 times PSMA expression particularly in high grade and variant tumor types.[53–58] In such patients, FDG PET-CT has an important role to play. Zhou and colleagues[59] shown that PSMA PET-CT performed better than FDG in primary staging while retrospectively analyzing 21 men with prostate cancer. A significant role of FDG PET-CT is in detecting high-grade prostate carcinoma where there is low-grade PSMA uptake because of dedifferentiation or neuroendocrine differentiation as has been shown by a study by Rosar and colleagues[60] while analyzing 66 males referred for radioligand therapy (RLT). They found 41/66 (62%) who had at least one PSMA-negative/FDG-positive lesion showed higher levels of neuroendocrine markers.

Restaging

Men with localized prostate cancer are treated with curative intent either with RP or RT after which there is lasting and complete response, especially in low-risk group; however, approximately 32% of patients will develop BCR within 10 years.[61] BCR is defined as: 0.2 ng/mL or higher with a second confirmatory increase after RP and increase of serum PSA > 2 ng/mL above nadir with negative conventional imaging.[4,62] Prostate carcinoma showing BCR is a spectrum of disease encompassing—hormone-sensitive non-metastatic, hormone-sensitive metastatic, and castrate-resistant metastatic cancer with newer therapeutic modalities (second-generation anti-androgens such as abiraterone and enzalutamide and newer taxane-based chemotherapy with docetaxel and cabazitaxel) has good initial response in the first two and the later showing a potentially lethal form of disease. In BCR scenario, 25% to 35% of cases show only local recurrence, 20% to 25% have distant metastases only, and 45% to 55% shows both.[63] RLT in advanced mCRPC is a novel therapeutic option and has shown promising results. Hence, it is imperative to diagnose recurrence early in the course to devise an effective treatment plan.

PSMA PET-CT scan shows higher tumor-to-background ratios and higher detection rates than choline PET-CT in BCR with low rise in serum PSA levels.[64] Afshar-Oromieh et al. in a large study over 319 patients with BCR reported that PSMA PET-CT detected at least one lesion in 83% of cases with excellent detection rates even at low PSA levels (detection rates of 50% with PSA < 0.5 ng/mL) and correlated with PSA levels and not with Gleason score and PSA doubling time (PSA DT).[65] Similar results were seen in another study comprising patients with BCR post RP, by the same group: overall detection rate was 89.5% and detection rates were higher with high PSA values being 96.8% at PSA 2 ng/mL or more and 57.9% with PSA of 0.5 to less than 0.2 ng/mL.[66] A meta-analysis by Perera and colleagues including 16 articles with a cumulative 1309 patients reported a pooled detection rate of 75% in patients with BCR and was superior to that with choline PET-CT showing overall detection rate of 62%.[67,68]

FDG PET-CT is an important imaging modality especially in advanced prostate cancer: high Gleason score and grade, high serum PSA, shorter PSA DT and variant tumor types, viz. neuroendocrine differentiated and ductal variant of prostate carcinoma and also poorly differentiated prostate carcinoma. In BCR, FDG PET-CT has limited utility and is useful in detecting osseous lesions particularly (can differentiate between active and dormant healed lesions), and in detecting high-grade transformation early during the course of disease. Chang and colleagues[69] in their study of 24 patients with PSA relapse after definitive treatment of localized prostate cancer, FDG PET detected nodal involvement in 75% of the patients with sensitivity, specificity, accuracy, positive predictive value (PPV), and negative predictive value (NPV) of FDG in detecting lymph nodal metastases in biochemical relapse was 75%, 100%, 83.3%, 100%, and 67.7%, respectively. Schoder and colleagues[70] in a retrospective study of 91 patients with PSA relapse post-prostatectomy showed that mean PSA level was higher in FDG PET-positive patients than FDG PET-negative patients; however, overall detection rate of local and systemic disease by FDG in PSA relapse was quite modest and reported as 31%. Other studies have shown FDG PET-CT to be particularly useful in imaging and staging of advanced prostate carcinoma with rising PSA levels despite treatment.[71,72] Richter and colleagues[73] while evaluating dual-tracer PET-CT using ^{11}C-choline and ^{18}F-FDG in 73 patients inferred: while sensitivity of ^{11}C-choline was higher than FDG latter correlated significantly with Gleason score.

Selection of Appropriate Therapeutic Modality

With advent and introduction of newer therapeutic modality in management of prostate carcinoma, particularly metastatic and castrate resistant states, appropriate therapeutic intervention at a particular stage in disease course holds critical importance. Newer anti-androgens such as abiraterone and enzalutamide and chemotherapeutic agents such as docetaxel and cabazitaxel, oligometastatic-targeted therapy, and RLT-targeting PSMA using $^{177}Lu/^{225}Ac$ have really strengthened the armamentarium against metastatic prostate cancer. Imaging, particularly functional imaging using PET-CT provides objective noninvasive evaluation of overall disease burden and tumor biology especially while using "dual-tracer" PET imaging targeting different aspects of tumor biology (viz. differentiation, proliferative status, etc.).

Basu and colleagues[73] in their editorial review discussed the role of "dual-tracer" PET-CT using PSMA and FDG-PET-CT and the results obtained, in devising a step-care management algorithm to individualize the available therapeutic alternatives in mCRPC setting. They recommended the use of taxane based chemotherapy (docetaxel and cabazitaxel) followed by ADT or vice versa in patients with FDG+/PSMA–, FDG+/PSMA+ and high Gleason score patients whereas RLT with or without ADT should be considered in patients with FDG-/PSMA + imaging and low Gleason score.[74]

PSMA PET-CT according to few current guidelines should be considered in high-risk and advanced prostate cancer at baseline before surgery (RP) or external beam radiotherapy (EBRT) and definitive curative treatment should be deferred.[49,51] PSMA PET-CT as baseline imaging modality detects nodal and skeletal metastases in 26.7% and 12.2%, respectively.[45] Oligometastatic directed therapy either using surgery and RT is a promising approach and warrants metastasis to be detected early; PSMA PET-CT in this regard will be useful for better control of disease.[75] Hofman and colleagues in their landmark single-center single-arm, phase 2 study studying 177Lu-PSMA radioligand treatment in patients with mCRPC (Lu-PSMA trial) selected patients with PSMA+/FDG-disease (based on "dual-tracer" PET-CT concept) and found good clinical outcome post 177Lu-PSMA therapy in this group (TheraP trial), whereas patients with FDG + disease were not considered for RLT and they showed rapid disease progression and worse clinical outcome.[76,77] Suman and colleagues[22] in their study evaluated the efficacy of ^{177}Lu-PSMA-617 PRLT in patients from a large tertiary cancer center recruiting aggressive and unselected cohort of mCRPC patients showed that high FDG SUVmax (>15) was associated with

higher chances of treatment failure. Fifteen patients showed FDG SUVmax > 15 and out them 12 patients (80%) showed progressive disease, whereas out of 22 patients with FDG SUVmax < 15, only nine patients (40%) had progressive disease.[22] Most of the published studies hence showed high FDG uptake to be an independent risk factor for disease progression and in predicting treatment failure, especially ^{177}Lu-PSMA PRLT (Fig. 3).

Treatment Response Evaluation

Treatment response evaluation in prostate cancer is done under following heads: symptomatic, biochemical, and imaging response (both functional and anatomic). Functional imaging response evaluation is done using FDG and PSMA/choline PET-CT, whereas anatomic imaging response is done using CT scan and MRI. PET-based functional imaging response evaluation is more objective and less interpreter dependent, whereas anatomic imaging using Response Evaluation Criteria in Solid Tumors (RECIST) 1.1 depends more on observer and in this way is less objective. Anatomic imaging depends more on morphologic assessment of lesions, is less quantitative, whereas functional imaging provides more quantitative assessment, conventionally in terms of standardized uptake value (SUV) and with introduction and use of newer and more elaborate PET quantitative parameters such as measured tumor volume (MTV), total lesion glycolysis (TLG for FDG), etc.

Studies have shown decrease in FDG accumulation in androgen-sensitive prostate cancer after ADT and hence potential role of FDG in response assessment and detection of failure of ADT in HSPCand development of castration resistant state early in the course.[78,79] FDG is also important in response assessment of osseous disease, especially in castration-resistant prostate cancer (CRPC) which is generally FDG concentrating and does not concentrate FDG when they are healed and inactive. Cecil and colleagues evaluated response using ^{11}C-Choline in men with mCRPC before and after chemotherapy (docetaxel) and Choline PET showed progressive disease in 44% of patients showing 50% or greater reduction in PSA levels inferring that choline PET could identify disease progression despite PSA response.[80] Other studies where Choline PET has been used for treatment response evaluation in mCRPC patients being treated with newer ADT (abiraterone and enzalutamide) have shown that it has prognostic implication in terms of PFS and OS.[81-83] PSMA PET-CT for response evaluation

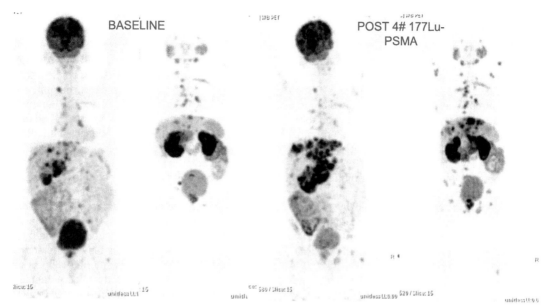

Fig. 3. Maximum intensity projection images of FDG and ⁶⁸Ga-PSMA PET-CT scans at baseline and after four cycles of ¹⁷⁷Lu-PSMA therapy of patient with mCRPC (Gleason score 3 + 4) with nodal, skeletal and visceral (hepatic) metastases, referred for ¹⁷⁷Lu-PSMA therapy after multiple lines of treatment failure (B/L orchidectomy, bicalutamide, Honvan, abiraterone, docetaxel, cabazitaxel, enzalutamide, and mitoxantrone). Patient had concordant PSMA and FDG avid disease and showed progression after four cycles of ¹⁷⁷Lu-PSMA therapy (serum PSA 1181 ng/mL after four cycles of ¹⁷⁷Lu-PSMA vs 237 ng/mL at baseline before ¹⁷⁷Lu-PSMA). Patient was then started on Nab-paclitaxel and carboplatin, received 28 cycles of the same with initial partial response followed by progression and culminating in death.

is recommended before and after any local or systemic therapy in patients at risk of having metastatic disease. Emmett and colleagues in their prospective study evaluating ADT on 15 men with both metastatic HSPC and mCRPC have shown decreased PSMA uptake in HSPC and increased PSMA (& decreased FDG) uptake in mCRPC post ADT.[84] In a recent study by Suman and colleagues evaluating clinical outcomes using "dual-tracer" PET-CT post 177Lu-PSMA RLT in mCRPC showed 43% to be responders (complete response (CR), partial response (PR) & stable disease (SD)) and 57% to be non-responders (progressive disease) and in combination therapy (with newer ADT - abiraterone) the response was seen in 78% of patients and 22% were non responders.[22,85] High FDG uptake predicts increased chances of treatment failure and in identifying non-responders at an early stage (see **Fig. 3**).

Prognostication

Recent studies have strongly suggested prognostic role of FDG PET-CT in prostate cancer, especially in high grade, advanced and castrate resistant disease; however, the same does not hold good for PSMA PET-CT and the available data is limited. Ferdinandus and colleagues while

studying for prognostic biomarkers in men with mCRPC receiving 177Lu-PSMA therapy inferred that high FDG SUVmax is associated with shorter survival and longer survival was associated with high intensity uptake on PSMA PET and low volume of FDG avid disease in patients treated with 177Lu-PSMA therapy.[86] Another recent study evaluating prognostic implication of dual-tracer PTE CT using PSMA and FDG have shown significantly shorter survival for patients with at least one FDG+/PSMA-lesion.[87] Lavallee and colleagues in their prospective study recruiting 148 consecutive patients with high Gleason score (≥8) found 66% of patients to show focal intra-prostatic FDG uptake.[88] They inferred that an FDG SUVmax ≥4.6 was statistically significantly associated with high Gleason score, extra-capsular extension, seminal vesicle invasion and lymph nodal metastases; also in the multivariate analysis intra-prostatic SUVmax ≥4.6 was associated with a two-fold increased risk of BCR in the year following surgery.[88] Also, patients with an intra-prostatic SUVmax ≥4.6 had estimated median BCR-free survival of 11.3 months as against 49.5 months for those with lower SUVmax and showed shorter time to castration resistance post RP.[88]

Jadvar and colleagues prospectively investigated 76 men with metastatic HSPC to predict time to hormonal treatment failure (THTF) with FDG PET-CT scan and showed 35% THTF probability at 5 years with all PET parameters significantly correlating with THTF and on multivariate analysis only sum of SUVmax and number of lesions significantly correlated with THTF.[89] When sum of SUVmax was grouped into quartile ranges, there was significantly worse survival probability for patients in fourth quartile range (7 months) than in the first (64 months).[89] Few of the recent studies have investigated FDG PET-CT for treatment response evaluation and found high FDG uptake to be associated with significantly worse survival outcomes and high probability of treatment failure (23, 89, 91, see **Fig. 3**). In recent study by Bauckneht and colleagues in their retrospective analysis to study prognostic potential of FDG PET-CT to estimate systemic treatment response duration in mCRPC patients found MTV as sole independent predictor of overall survival (OS) and PSA & TLG as independent predictors of treatment response duration.[90] Furthermore, lower TLG was significantly associated with higher treatment success rates for androgen receptor targeting agents (particularly abiraterone and enzalutamide).[90]

DISCUSSION

Dual/Multi tracer PET-CT is an evolving concept in non-invasively characterizing tumor biology and has been successfully used in management of NET where somatostatin receptor (SSTR) PET and FDG PET is routinely used in personalized decision making in addition to Ki-67/Mib-1 labeling index.[20,21,91] As the recent studies have shown PSMA PET-CT to be better performing than PET-CT targeting choline and dihydrotestosterone (DHT) for prostate cancer and the available data on these PET tracers are also not that robust, in this review we meant PSMA and FDG with dual-tracer. The role of dual/multi tracer PET-CT in prostate cancer is still in its infantile stage but initial results are encouraging.

Dual-tracer PET-CT using PSMA and FDG in prostate cancer, particularly has a role in high Gleason score, aggressive, metastatic and castration resistant disease with shorter PSA DT for baseline staging, restaging, selection of appropriate treatment modality, treatment response evaluation and prognostication, predicting overall & progression free survival and treatment response duration as has been elaborated in earlier sections. In a recently published study, Adnan and Basu proposed a six-tier dual-tracer PET-CT scoring system in mCRPC patients using PSMA and FDG PET-CT (Pro-PET score) (24, see **Fig. 1**). The authors found that Pro-PET score

statistically significantly correlated with response (symptomatic, biochemical, anatomic & functional responses) and with outcome (overall and progression free survival) after ^{177}Lu-PSMA-617 therapy.[23] Furthermore, "Pro-PET" scoring could potentially select patients who will benefit from 177Lu-PSMA therapy either as mono therapy or in combination therapy and in whom chemotherapy and other treatment modalities should be considered (24, **Fig. 2**).

Another potential area where PET-CT could be of particular importance in prostate cancer, especially PET-CT in regional and distant recurrence for early detection and oligometastases directed therapeutic approach. Ost and colleagues in their systemic review of metastatic directed therapy in locoregional and distant metastases underscored the role of PET-CT scan for early detection of patients who can benefit from oligometastases directed therapy.[75] Wang and colleagues in a single arm prospective trial on 37 men with high-risk early CRPC found that among 30% of the men with no PSMA uptake, 27% (8% overall) showed metastatic disease on FDG PET, thereby use of "dual-tracer" PET improved the detection of metastatic disease from 65% to 73% with negative conventional imaging.[92] Another retrospective case control study in 72 patients with BCR post-RP showed FDG PET-positive lesions in 17% patients with negative PSMA PET-CT and high Gleason score ($\geq$8).[93] Also 5% to 10% patients with primary prostate cancer have low PSMA activity which evades detection by PSMA PET-CT mostly in high grade (Gleason grade group) and variant tumor types where FDG PET has some role to play in terms of disease detection.[53–58] Furthermore, PSMA PET-CT in addition to its high sensitivity has a negative likelihood ratio of 0.05 which translates to a 20-fold decrease in odds of prostate carcinoma being present in patients with negative PSMA PET, thereby making PSMA PET-CT a potential rule out test in patients with clinical and biochemical findings suspicious for prostate cancer and hence avoid unnecessary biopsies.[26] "Dual-tracer" PET-CT in this way (using FDG and PSMA) evaluates prostate carcinoma with most possible aspects to provide comprehensive insights into tumor biology and hence is effective in devising curated personalized treatment strategy (see **Fig. 3**). In present era of multiple therapeutic options, particularly for mCRPC, "dual-tracer" PET effectively selects patients who will have maximum benefit with PSMA targeting RLT as mono-therapy or combination therapy and to exclude the patients who will not benefit from the radionuclide therapy and to be considered upfront for alternative therapeutic options.[23,76,77]

SUMMARY

Dual-tracer PET-CT in prostate carcinoma is a rapidly evolving concept with encouraging results as in terms of an overall analysis of tumor biology: PSMA PET-CT is very sensitive and specific modality for detection of prostate-specific disease and guide treatment, whereas FDG PET in prostate carcinoma identifies: (a) disease negative on PSMA PET-CT, (b) osseous metastases, (c) gives measure of tumor glycolysis and aggressive tumor behavior, (d) raises suspicion of aggressive and variant tumor types, and (e) identifies lesions for targeted biopsies to characterize biological and molecular heterogeneity depending on imaging discordance. Dual-tracer PET-CT, hence, should be considered in all patients with high Gleason grade group, negative PSMA PET-CT, shorter PSA DT and in castrate resistant cases for timely and effective triage of patients for available treatment options especially PSMA targeting RLT using ^{177}Lu/^{225}Ac.

DISCLOSURE

The authors have nothing to disclose.

REFERENCES

1. Siegel RL, Miller KD, Jemal A. Cancer statistics, 2020. CA Cancer J Clin 2020;70:7–30.
2. SEER stat fact sheets: prostate. National Cancer Institute. Available at: http://seer.cancer.gov/statfacts/html/prost.html. Accessed 5 June 2013.
3. D'Amico AV, Moul J, Carroll PR, et al. Cancer-specific mortality after surgery or radiation for patients with clinically localized prostate cancer managed during the prostate-specific antigen era. J Clin Oncol 2003; 21:2163–72.
4. Scher HI, Halabi S, Tannock I, et al. Design and end points of clinical trials for patients with progressive prostate cancer and castrate levels of testosterone: recommendations of the ProstateCancer Clinical Trials Working Group. J Clin Oncol 2008;26:1148–59 [PubMed: 18309951].
5. Fox JJ, Morris MJ, Larson SM, et al. Developing imaging strategies for castrationresistant prostate cancer. Acta Oncol (Madr) 2011;50(suppl 1):39–48.
6. Chen Y, Sawyers CL, Scher HI. Targeting the androgen receptor pathway in prostate cancer. Curr Opin Pharmacol 2008;8(4):440–8.
7. Han M, Partin AW, Pound CR, et al. Long-termbiochemical disease-free and cancer-specific survival following anatomic radical retropubic prostatectomy. The 15-year Johns Hopkins experience. Urol Clin North Am 2001;28:555–65.
8. Joniau S, Briganti A, Gontero P, et al. Stratification of high-riskprostate cancer into prognostic categories: a European multi- institutional study. Eur Urol 2015; 67:157–64.
9. Bolla M, vanPoppel H, Tombal B, et al. Postoperative radiotherapyafter radical prostatectomy for high-risk prostate cancer: long-term results of a randomised controlled trial (EORTC trial 22911). Lancet 2012; 380:2018–27.
10. Shariat SF, Kattan MW, Vickers AJ, et al. Critical review of prostate cancer predictive tools. Future Oncol 2009;5:1555–84.
11. Briganti A, Karnes RJ, Gandaglia G, et al. Natural history of surgicallytreated high-risk prostate cancer. Urol Oncol 2015;33. Error: Page (1631e7) is higher than LPage (13)!.
12. Ploussard G, Masson-Lecomte A, Beauval JB, et al. Radical prostatectomy for high-riskprostatecancerdefinedby preoperativecriteria: oncologicfollow-upinnational multicenterstudyin813-patientsand assessment of easy-to-useprognostic substratification. Urology 2011;78:607–13.
13. Ryan CJ, Smith MR, de Bono JS, et al. Abiraterone inmetastatic prostate cancer withoutprevious chemotherapy. N Englj Med 2013;368:13848.
14. Beer TM, Armstrong AJ, Rathkopf DE, et al. Enzalutamide in metastatic prostate cancer beforechemotherapy. N Engl J Med 2014;371:424–33.
15. Tannock IF, de Wit R, Berry WR, et al. Docetaxel plus prednisone or mitoxantrone plus prednisonefor advanced prostate cancer. N Engl J Med 2004; 351:1502–12.
16. Berthold DR, Pond GR, Soban F, et al. Docetaxel plus prednisone or mitoxantrone plus prednisone for advanced prostate cancer: updated survival in the TAX327 study. J Clin Oncol official J theAmerican Soc Clin Oncol 2008;26:242–5.
17. de Bono JS, Oudard S, Ozguroglu M, et al. Prednisone plus cabazitaxel or mitoxantrone formetastatic castration-resistant prostate cancer progressing after docetaxel treatment: a randomised open-label trial. Lancet (London,England) 2010;376:1147–54.
18. Kim YJ, Kim YI. Therapeutic responses and survival effects of177Lu-PSMA-617 Radioligand therapy in metastatic castrateresistant prostate cancer: a meta-analysis. Clin Nucl Med 2018;43:728–34.
19. Pouliot F, Johnson M, Wu L. Non-invasive molecular imaging of prostate cancer lymph node metastasis. Trends Mol Med 2009;15:254–62.
20. Basu S, Sirohi B, Shrikhande SV. Dual-tracer imaging approach inassessing tumor biology and heterogeneity in neuroendocrine tu- mors: its correlation with tumor proliferation index and possible multifaceted implications for personalized clinical management decisions, with focus on PRRT. Eur J Nucl Med Mol Imaging 2014;41(8):1492–6.
21. Basu S, Ranade R, Thapa P. Correlation and discordance of tumourproliferation index and molecular imaging characteristics and their implications for

treatment decisions and outcome pertaining to peptide receptor radionuclide therapy in patients with advanced neurondocrinetumour: developing a personalized model. Nucl Med Commun 2015; 36(8):766–74.

22. Suman S, Parghane RV, Joshi A, et al. Therapeutic efficacy, prognostic variables and clinical outcome of (177)Lu-PSMA-617 PRLT in progressive mCRPC follow- ing multiple lines of treatment: prognostic implications of high FDG uptake on dual-tracer PET-CT vis-à-vis Gleason Score in such cohort. Br J Radiol 2019;10:20190380.

23. Adnan A, Basu S. Concept proposal for a six-tier integrated dual-tracer PET-CT (68Ga-PSMA and FDG) image scoring system ('Pro-PET' score) and examining its potential implications in metastatic castration-resistant prostate carcinoma theranostics and prognosis. Nucl Med Commun 2021;42(5):566–74.

24. Ahmed HU, El-Shater Bosaily A, Brown LC, et al. Diagnostic accuracy of multi-parametric MRI and TRUS biopsy in prostate cancer (PROMIS): a paired validating confirmatory study. Lancet 2017; 389(10071):815–22.

25. Kwan Timothy N, et al. Performance of Ga-68 PSMA PET/CT for diagnosis and grading of local prostate cancer. Prostate Int 2021;9(2):107–12.

26. Satapathy S, Singh H, Kumar R, et al. Diagnostic accuracy of 68Ga-PSMA PET/CT for initial detection in patients with suspected prostate cancer: a systematic review and meta-analysis. AJR Am J Roentgenol 2021;216(3):599–607.

27. Jadvar H. Is there use for FDG-PET in prostate cancer? Semin Nucl Med 2016;46(6):502–6.

28. Sahin E, Elboga U, Kalender E, et al. Clinical significance of incidental FDG uptake in theprostategland detected by PET/CT. Int J Clin Exp Med 2015;8: 10577–85.

29. Bertagna F, Sadeghi R, Giovanella L, et al. Incidental uptake of 18F-fluorodeoxyglucose intheprostate gland. Systematic review and meta-analysis on prevalence and risk ofmalignancy. Nuklearmedizin 2014;53:249–58.

30. Brown AM, Lindenberg ML, Sankineni S, et al. Does focal incidental 18F-FDG uptake in theprostate gland have significance? Abdom Imaging 2015;40: 3222–9.

31. Kang PM, Seo WI, Lee SS, et al. Incidental abnormal FDG uptake in the prostate on 18-fluoro-2-deoxyglucose positron emission tomography-computed tomography. Asian Pac J Cancer Prev 2014;15: 8699–703.

32. Seino H, Ono S, Miura H, et al. Incidental prostate 18F-FDG uptake without calcification indicates possibility of prostate cancer. Oncol Rep 2014;31: 1517–22.

33. Hwang I, Chong A, Jung SI, et al. Is further evaluation needed for incidental focal uptake in the prostate in 18-fluoro-2-deoxyglucose positron emission tomography-computed tomography images? Ann Nucl Med 2013;27(2):140–5.

34. Awwad HM, Geisel J, Obeid R. The role of choline in prostatecancer. Clin Biochem 2012;45:1548–53.

35. Muller SA, Holzapfel K, Seidl C, et al. Characterization of choline uptake inprostate cancer cells following bicalutamide anddocetaxel treatment. Eur J Nucl Med Mol Imaging 2009;36:1434–42.

36. Oka S, Hattori R, Kurosaki F, et al. A preliminary study ofanti-1-amino-3-18Ffluorocyclobutyl-1-carboxylic acid for the detection of prostate cancer. J Nucl Med 2007;48:46–55.

37. Sasajima T, Ono T, Shimada N, et al. Trans-1-amino-3-18F-fluorocyclobutanecarboxylic acid(anti-18F-FACBC) is a feasiblealternative to 11C-methyl-L-methionine and magnetic resonanceimaging for monitoring treatment response in gliomas. Nucl Med Biol 2013;40:808–15.

38. Oka S, Okudaira H, Yoshida Y, et al. Transport mechanisms oftrans-1-amino-3-fluoro[1(14)C] cyclobutanecarboxylic acid in prostate cancer cells. Nucl Med Biol 2012;39:109–19.

39. Schuster DM, Nanni C, Fanti S. PET tracers beyond FDG in prostatecancer. Semin Nucl Med 2016;46: 507–21.

40. Savir-Baruch B, Zanoni L, Schuster DM. Imaging of prostate cancerusing fluciclovine. PET Clin 2017; 12:145–57.

41. Fowler JE Jr, Sanders J, Bigler SA, et al. Percent free prostate specific antigen and cancer detection in black and white men with total prostate specific antigen 2.5 to 9.9 ng./ml. J Urol 2000;163(5): 1467–70.

42. Hövels AM, Heesakkers RA, Adang EM, et al. The diagnosticaccuracy of CT and MRI in the staging of pelvic lymph nodes in patients with prostate cancer: a meta-analysis. Clin Radiol 2008;63(4):387–95.

43. American Urological Association. AUA guidelines. American Urological Association website. Available at: http://www.auanet.org/guidelines.

44. National Comprehensive Cancer Network. Recent updatesto NCCN clinical practice guidelines in oncology (NCCN Guidelines®): prostate cancer—version 1.2017. National Comprehensive Cancer Network website. Available at: https://www.nccn.org/professionals/physician_gls/recently_updated.asp. Accessed January 12, 2017.

45. Mottet N, Bellmunt J, Briers E, et al. EAU prostate cancerguidelines 2017. European Association of Urology website. Available at: http://uroweb.org/guidelineprostate-cancer/. Accessed June 1, 2017.

46. Uprimny C, Kroiss AS, Decristoforo C, et al. 68Ga-PSMA-11PET/CT in primary staging of prostate cancer: PSA and Gleason score predict the intensity of tracer accumulation in the primary tumour. Eur J Nucl Med Mol Imaging 2017;44(6):941–9.

47. Fendler WP, Schmidt DF, Wenter V, et al. 68Ga-PSMA PET/CT detects the location and extent of primary prostate cancer. J Nucl Med 2016;57(11):1720–5.

48. Giesel FL, Sterzing F, Schlemmer HP, et al. Intra-individualcomparison of 68Ga-PSMA-11-PET/CT and multi-parametric MR for imaging of primary prostate cancer. Eur J Nucl Med Mol Imaging 2016;43(8):1400–6.

49. Fendler WP, Eiber M, Beheshti M, et al. 68Ga-PSMA PET/CT: joint EANM and SNMMI procedure guideline for prostate cancer imaging—version 1.0. Eur J Nucl Med Mol Imaging 2017;44(6):1014–24.

50. Litwin MS, Tan HJ. The diagnosis and treatment ofprostate cancer. J Am Med Assoc 2017;317(24):2532–42.

51. Hofman MS, Lawrentschuk N, Francis RJ, et al. Prostate-specific membrane antigen PET-CT in patients with high-risk prostate cancer before curative-intent surgery or radiotherapy (proPSMA): a prospective, randomised, multicentre study. The Lancet 2020;395(10231):1208–16.

52. Donato P, Roberts MJ, Morton A, et al. Improved specificitywith 68Ga PSMA PET/CT to detect clinically significant lesions "invisible" on multiparametric MRI of the prostate: a single institution comparative analysis with radical prostatectomy histology. Eur J Nucl Med Mol Imaging 2019;46(1):20–30.

53. Maurer T, Eiber M, Schwaiger M, et al. Current use of PSMA-PET in prostate cancer management. Nat Rev Urol 2016;13(4):226–35.

54. Roberts MJ, Morton A, Donato A, et al. 68Ga-PSMA PET/CT tumour intensity pre-operatively predicts adverse path- ological outcomes and progression-free survival in localised prostate cancer. Eur J Nucl Med Mol Imaging 2021;48(2):477–82.

55. Lengana T, Lawal IO, Boshomane TG, et al. 68Ga-PSMAPET/CT replacing bone scan in the initial staging of skeletal metastasis in prostate cancer: a fait accompli? Clin Genitourinary Cancer 2018;16(5):392–401.

56. Demirci E, Sahin OE, Ocak M, et al. Normal distribution pattern and physiological variants of 68Ga-PSMA-11 PET/CT imaging. Nucl Med Commun 2016;37(11):1169–79.

57. Ghosh A, Heston WDW. Tumor target prostatespecific membrane antigen (PSMA) and its regulation in prostate cancer. J Cell Biochem 2004;91(3):528–39.

58. Chakraborty PS, Tripathi M, Agarwal KK, et al. Metastatic poorly differentiated prostatic carcinoma with neuroendocrine differentiation. Clin Nucl Med 2015;40(2):e163–6.

59. Zhou X, Li Y, Jiang X, et al. Intra-individual comparison of18F-PSMA-1007 and 18F-FDG PET/CT in the evaluation of patients with prostate cancer. Front Oncol 2020;10:585213.

60. Rosar F, Ribbat K, Ries M, et al. Neuron-specific enolasehas potential value as a biomarker for [18F]FDG/[68Ga]Ga- PSMA-11 PET mismatch findings in advanced mCRPC patients. EJNMMI Res 2020;10(1).

61. Roehl KA, Han M, Ramos CG, et al. Cancer progression and survival rates following anatomical radical retropubic prostatectomy in 3,478 consecutive patients: long-term results. J Urol 2004;172(3):910–4.

62. Roach M 3rd, Hanks G, Thames H Jr, et al. Defining biochemical failure following radiotherapy with or without hormonal therapy in men with clinically localized prostate cancer: recommendations of the RTOG-ASTRO Phoenix Consensus Conference. Int J Radiat Oncol Biol Phys 2006;65(4):965–74.

63. Carroll P. Rising PSA after a radical treatment. Eur Urol 2001;40(2):9–16.

64. Afshar-Oromieh A, Zechmann CM, Malcher A, et al. Comparison of PET imaging with a 68Ga-labelled PSMA ligand and 18F-choline-based PET/CT for the diagnosis of recurrent prostate cancer. Eur J Nucl Med Mol Imaging 2014;41(1):11–20.

65. Afshar-Oromieh A, Avtzi E, Giesel FL, et al. The diagnosticvalue of PET/CT imaging with the 68Ga-labelled PSMA ligand HBED-CC in the diagnosis of recurrent prostate cancer. Eur J Nucl Med Mol Imaging 2015;42(2):197–209.

66. Eiber M, Maurer T, Souvatzoglou M, et al. Evaluation ofhybrid 68Ga-PSMA ligand PET/CT in 248 patients with biochemical recurrence after radical prostatectomy. J Nucl Med 2015;56(5):668–74.

67. Perera M, Papa N, Christidis D, et al. Sensitivity, specificity,and predictors of positive 68Ga–prostate-specific membrane antigen positron emission tomography in advanced prostate cancer: a systematic review and meta-analysis. Eur Urol 2016;70(6):926–37.

68. Fanti S, Minozzi S, Castellucci P, et al. PET/CT with 11C-choline for evaluation of prostate cancer patients with biochemical recurrence: meta-analysis and critical review of available data. Eur J Nucl Med Mol Imaging 2016;43(1):55–69.

69. Chang CH, Wu HC, Tsai JJP, et al. Detecting metastatic pelvic lymph nodes by (18)F-2-deoxyglucose positron emission tomography in patients with prostate-specific antigen relapse after treatment for localized prostate cancer. Urol Int 2003;70:311–5.

70. Schöder H, Herrmann K, Gönen M, et al. 2-[18F]fluoro-2-deoxyglucose positron emission tomography for detection of disease in patients with prostate-specific antigen relapse after radical prostatectomy. Clin Cancer Res 2005;11:4761–9.

71. Sanz G, Robles JE, Giménez M, et al. Positron emission tomography with 18fluorine-labelled deoxyglucose: utility in localized and advanced prostate cancer. BJU Int 1999;84:1028–31.

72. Sung J, Espiritu JI, Segall GM, et al. Fluorodeoxyglucose positron emission tomography studies in the

diagnosis and staging of clinically advanced prostate cancer. BJU Int 2003;92:24–7.

73. Richter JA, Rodríguez M, Rioja J, et al. Dual-tracer 11C-choline and FDG-PET in the diagnosis of biochemical prostate cancer relapse after radical treatment. Mol Imaging Biol 2010;12(2):210–7.

74. Basu S, Parghane RV, Suman S, et al. Towards personalizing treatment strategies in mCRPC: can dual-tracer PET-CT provide insights into tumor biology, guide the optimal treatment sequence, and individualize decision-making (between chemotherapy, second-generation anti-androgens and PSMA-directed radioligand therapy) early in the disease course? Eur J Nucl Med Mol Imaging 2020; 47(8):1793–7.

75. Ost P, Bossi A, Decaestecker K, et al. Metastasis-directed therapy of regional and distant recurrences after curative treatment of prostate cancer: a systematic review of the literature. Eur Urol 2015; 67(5):852–63.

76. Hofman MS, Violet J, Hicks RJ, et al. [177Lu]-PSMA-617 radionuclide treatment in patients with metastatic castration-resistant prostate cancer (LuPSMA trial): a single-centre, single-arm, phase 2 study. Lancet Oncol 2018;19(6):825–33.

77. Hofman MS, Emmett L, Sandhu S, et al. [177Lu]Lu-PSMA-617 versus cabazitaxel in patients with metastatic castration-resistant prostate cancer (TheraP): a randomised, open-label, phase 2 trial. Lancet 2021;397(10276):797–804.

78. Oyama N, Akino H, Suzuki Y, et al. FDG PET for evaluating the change of glucose metabolism in prostate cancer after androgen ablation. Nucl Med Commun 2001;22(9):963–9.

79. Jadvar H, Xiankui L, Shahinian A, et al. Glucose metabolism of human prostate cancer mouse xenografts. Mol Imaging 2005;4(2):91–7.

80. Ceci F, Castellucci P, Graziani T, et al. 11C-Choline PET/CT in castration-resistant prostate cancer patients treated with docetaxel. Eur J Nucl Med Mol Imaging 2016;43(1):84–91.

81. Maines F, Caffo O, Donner D, et al. Serial 18F-choline-PET imaging in patients receiving enzalutamide for metastatic castration-resistant prostate cancer: response assessment and imaging biomarkers. Future Oncol 2016;12(3):333–42.

82. De Giorgi U, Caroli P, Scarpi E, et al. 18F-Fluorocholine PET/CT for early response assessment in patients with metastatic castration-resistant prostate cancer treated with enzalutamide. Eur J Nucl Med Mol Imaging 2015;42(8):1276–83 [Published correction appears in Eur J Nucl Med Mol Imaging 2015; 42(8):1337–1338.].

83. De Giorgi U, Caroli P, Burgio SL, et al. Early outcome prediction on 18F-fluorocholine PET/CT in metastatic castration- resistant prostate cancer patients treated with abiraterone. Oncotarget 2014;5(23):12448–58.

84. Emmett LM, Yin C, Crumbaker M, et al. Rapid modulation of PSMA expression by androgen deprivation: serial 68Ga PSMA-11 PET in men with hormone sensitive and castrate resistant prostate cancer commencing androgen blockade. J Nucl Med 2018;118:223099. jnumed.

85. Suman S, Parghane RV, Joshi A, et al. Combined 177 Lu-PSMA-617 PRLT and abiraterone acetate versus 177 Lu-PSMA-617 PRLT monotherapy in metastatic castration-resistant prostate cancer: an observational study comparing the response and durability. Prostate 2021;81(15):1225–34.

86. Ferdinandus J, Violet J, Sandhu S, et al. Prognostic biomarkers in men with metastatic castration-resistant prostate cancer receiving [177Lu]-PSMA-617. Eur J Nucl Med Mol Imaging 2020;47(10): 2322–7.

87. Michalski K, Ruf J, Goetz C, et al. Prognostic implications of dual-tracer PET/CT: PSMA ligand and [18F]FDG PET/CT in patients undergoing [177Lu] PSMA radioligand therapy. Eur J Nucl Med Mol Imaging 2021;48(6):2024–30.

88. Lavallée E, Bergeron M, Buteau FA, et al. Increased prostate cancer glucose metabolism detected by 18F-fluorodeoxyglucose positron emission tomography/computed tomography in localised Gleason 8-10 prostate cancers identifies very high-risk patients for early recurrence and resistance to castration. Eur Urol Focus 2019;5(6):998–1006.

89. Jadvar H, Velez EM, Desai B, et al. Prediction of time to hormonal treatment failure in metastatic castration-sensitive prostate cancer with 18F-FDG PET/CT. J Nucl Med 2019;60(11):1524–30.

90. Bauckneht M, Bertagna F, Donegani MI, et al. The prognostic power of 18F-FDG PET/CT extends to estimating systemic treatment response duration in metastatic castration-resistant prostate cancer (mCRPC) patients. Prostate Cancer Prostatic Dis 2021;24(4):1198–207.

91. Adnan A, Basu S. Discordance between Histopathological grading and Dual-tracer PET-CT findings (68Ga-DOTATATE and FDG) in metastatic Neuroendocrine Neoplasms and outcome of 177Lu-DOTATATE PRRT: does in-vivo molecular PET imaging perform better from 'prediction of tumour biology' viewpoint? [published online ahead of print, 2021 Dec 7]. J Nucl Med Technol 2021;121:261998.

92. Wang B, Liu C, Wei Y, et al. A prospective trial of 68Ga-PSMA and 18F-FDG PET/CT in nonmetastatic prostate cancer patients with an early PSA progression during castration. Clin Cancer Res 2020;26(17): 4551–8.

93. Chen R, Wang Y, Shi Y, et al. Diagnostic value of (18) F-FDG PET/CT in patients with biochemical recurrent prostate cancer and negative (68)Ga-PSMA PET/CT. Eur J Nucl Med Mol Imaging 2021;48(9): 2970–7.

Assessing Coronary Artery and Aortic Calcification in Patients with Prostate Cancer Using ^{18}F-Sodium Fluoride PET/Computed Tomography

William Y. Raynor, MD[a,b], Austin J. Borja, BA[a], Vincent Zhang, BA[a],
Esha Kothekar, MD[a], Hui Chong Lau, MD[c], Sze Jia Ng, MD[c],
Siavash Mehdizadeh Seraj, MD[a], Chaitanya Rojulpote, MD[a],
Raheleh Taghvaei, MD[a], Kevin Yu Jin, MD[a], Thomas J. Werner, MSE[a],
Poul Flemming Høilund-Carlsen[d,e],
Abass Alavi, MD, MD (Hon), PhD (Hon), DSc (Hon)[a],
Mona-Elisabeth Revheim, MD, PhD, MHA[a,f,g,h],*

KEYWORDS

- PET/CT • NaF • Microcalcification • Global assessment • Atherosclerosis
- Coronary artery disease • Angina pectoris

KEY POINTS

- ^{18}F-fluorodeoxyglucose (FDG) uptake reflects inflammation in the context of atherosclerosis mainly due to increased glycolysis by activated macrophages. However, FDG avidity is nonspecific and can be related to physiologic activity as well as other causes of infection, inflammation, and malignancy.
- ^{18}F-sodium fluoride (NaF) localizes to areas of active microcalcification and has been proposed as a sensitive and specific marker of atherogenic activity.
- To overcome difficulties in assessing atheromas due to the limited spatial resolution of PET, global quantification is necessary to determine overall disease activity.

Trial registration: NCT01724749.
[a] Department of Radiology, Hospital of the University of Pennsylvania, 3400 Spruce Street, Philadelphia, PA 19104, USA; [b] Department of Radiology, Rutgers Robert Wood Johnson Medical School, 1 Robert Wood Johnson Place, MEB #404, New Brunswick, NJ 08901, USA; [c] Department of Medicine, Crozer-Chester Medical Center, 1 Medical Center Boulevard, Upland, PA 19013, USA; [d] Department of Nuclear Medicine, Odense University Hospital, 5000 Odense C, Denmark; [e] Department of Clinical Research, University of Southern Denmark, 5000 Odense C, Denmark; [f] Division of Radiology and Nuclear Medicine, Oslo University Hospital, Sognsvannsveien 20, 0372 Oslo, Norway; [g] Institute of Clinical Medicine, Faculty of Medicine, University of Oslo, Problemveien 7, 0315 Oslo, Norway; [h] Division of Radiology and Nuclear Medicine, Postbox 4950, Nydalen, Oslo 0424, Norway
* Corresponding author. Division of Radiology and Nuclear Medicine, Postbox 4950, Nydalen, Oslo 0424, Norway
E-mail address: mona.elisabeth.revheim@ous-hf.no
Twitter: pfhc@rsyd.dk (P.F.H.-C.)

PET Clin 17 (2022) 653–659
https://doi.org/10.1016/j.cpet.2022.07.009

INTRODUCTION

Atherosclerosis is a cardiovascular disease characterized by the accumulation of lipid-derived inflammatory lesions on the inner arterial lumen. Cytokines produced by damaged endothelial cells promote the formation of a calcified fibrous cap composed of vascular smooth muscle. The calcification and subsequent arterial narrowing are significant causes of morbidity and mortality worldwide.[1] Coronary artery and aortic involvement in atherosclerosis has been extensively characterized and is believed to be heavily involved in obstructive cardiovascular diseases, such as pulmonary embolism, myocardial infarction, and stroke.[2] It has been understood for decades that atherosclerosis shares many molecular pathways with cancer, including alterations in the G1/S checkpoint and integrin/cadherin pathways, and atherosclerosis represents serious comorbidity within patients with cancer.[3,4] Therefore, early detection of atherosclerotic microcalcification within patients with cancer may facilitate the development and validation of anti-atherosclerotic drug therapy to treat this comorbidity.

Atherosclerotic changes may be detected through a number of imaging modalities. For example, an echocardiogram can create either two- or three-dimensional constructions of the cardiac vasculature.[5] Alternatively, MRI and computed tomography (CT) use magnetic field changes and X-rays, respectively, to generate three-dimensional representations of the affected vessels.[6] In contrast to these modalities, PET/ CT may be used to visualize atherosclerotic disease earlier in its progression on the molecular scale before macroscopic changes are evident.

[18]F-fluorodeoxyglucose (FDG)-PET/CT has been used extensively to detect inflammatory processes including atherosclerotic disease activity. However, recent studies have suggested that ^{18}F-sodium fluoride (NaF)-PET may be a more sensitive and specific tracer for the detection of atherosclerotic activity, and specifically, microcalcification.[7,8] NaF-PET/CT has most commonly been implicated in bone uptake, and there has been some evidence supporting NaF-PET/CT in the diagnosis of bone metastases.[9–11] Several preliminary studies have examined the role of NaF-PET/CT in atherosclerosis imaging with promising results regarding its superior ability to characterize active vascular microcalcification.[12–38] However, few studies have examined the role of NaF-PET/CT in the detection of cardiovascular disease in patients with cancer.

Thus, to improve understanding of the relationship between atherosclerotic disease and cancer, the goals of this study were to assess the feasibility of NaF-PET/CT to detect aortic and coronary artery atherosclerosis and to assess and compare NaF uptake in the aorta and coronary arteries of patients with prostate cancer, healthy control subjects, and patients with angina pectoris.

MATERIALS AND METHODS
Patient Population

Retrospective data from all male patients with prostate cancer and full-body NaF-PET/CT imaging performed at the Hospital of the University of Pennsylvania between January 2011 and May 2015 were included in this study. The study was approved by the University of Pennsylvania Institutional Review Board, and all work was performed in compliance with the Health Insurance Portability and Accountability Act (HIPAA).

Data from 33 healthy subjects and 33 patients with angina pectoris most similar in age to the patients with prostate cancer out of 139 subjects from the prospective Cardiovascular Molecular Calcification Assessed by NaF-PET/CT (CAMONA) study were analyzed. The CAMONA study was approved by the Danish National Committee on Biomedical Research Ethics, registered at ClinicalTrials.gov (NCT01724749), and conducted from 2012 to 2016, in compliance with the Declaration of Helsinki. Volunteers were recruited from the general population by local advertisement, as well as from the blood bank at Odense University Hospital, Denmark. Written informed consent was received from all subjects before the study. Subjects who had a history of cardiovascular disease, malignant neoplasm, deep vein thrombosis, pulmonary embolism, physical or mental disability, known immunodeficient state, or autoimmune disease were excluded.

Image Acquisition

All NaF-PET/CT scans were performed on hybrid PET/CT scanners 90 min after 3.0 MBq/kg intravenously injection of NaF radiotracer with an acquisition time of 2.5 min/bed position. For patients with prostate cancer, NaF-PET/CT imaging was performed on PET/CT scanners at the Hospital of the University of Pennsylvania (Gemini TF; Philips Healthcare, Best, The Netherlands) and for subjects from the CAMONA study, NaF-PET/CT imaging was performed at the Odense University Hospital (GE Discovery RX, STE, and 690/710 imaging systems; GE Healthcare, Milwaukee, WI, USA). The PET/CT scans were acquired in accordance with international guidelines, which include quality control, calibration and harmonization of the scanners, and standardized uptake value

(SUV) calculations.[39] PET images were reconstructed with iterative algorithms (Ordered Subset Expectation Maximization, OSEM). Low-dose CT was performed for anatomical correlation and attenuation correction. PET images were corrected for scattering, random coincidences, and scanner dead time.

Image Analysis

OsiriX MD software v.7.04 (DICOM viewer and image-analysis program, Pixmeo SARL; Bernex, Switzerland) was used to analyze the NaF-PET/CT images. Manual regions of interest (ROIs) were delineated on fused PET/CT images to measure global uptake in the coronary arteries, ascending aorta, aortic arch, and descending aorta. Global mean SUV (SUVmean) was calculated as the average value of all voxels in the ROI.

For the aortic arch, an ROI was manually delineated around the outer boundary of the artery on every PET/CT axial slice, starting at the most inferior slice in which the ascending and descending aorta are morphologically continuous and ending at the most superior slice that contains the aorta. To quantify the ascending and descending aorta, ROIs around the vessel boundary were delineated on every slice starting from the inferior-most slice of the aortic arch to the superior limit of the heart or the bifurcation into the iliac arteries, respectively. Coronary NaF uptake was measured by manually delineating an ROI around the cardiac silhouette, not including the aortic wall or aortic valves, on each axial PET/CT image.[40]

To determine global calcification activity in the structures of interest, the global mean standardized uptake value (SUVmean), defined as the average NaF uptake of all the voxels in the ROI, was determined. The target-to-background ratio (TBR) was determined by dividing the global SUVmean by the average NaF activity within an $1125 mm^3$ circular section of abdominal fat.[41]

Statistical Analysis

STATA software (Stata/IC Version 10.1, StataCorp, College Station, TX, USA) was used to perform all statistical analyses. Differences between TBR in subject groups were examined by two-tailed t-tests. Multivariable adjustment for age and sex was performed using multiple regressions. A value of $p < 0.05$ was considered significant.

RESULTS

The patients with prostate cancer included 33 men with an average age of 70 ± 6.6 years, the healthy subjects consisted of 16 men and 17 women with an average age of 59 ± 5.2 years, and patients with angina pectoris included 13 men and 20 women with an average age of 64 ± 5.0 years. TBR was compared between patients with prostate cancer, healthy subjects, and patients with angina pectoris (**Fig. 1**). Without multivariable adjustments, patients with cancer were observed to show a significant increase in TBR compared with healthy subjects in the coronary arteries (cancer = 5.3 ± 2.1; healthy = 4.2 ± 1.4; $p = 0.01$), ascending aorta (cancer = 6.6 ± 2.4; healthy = 5.4 ± 1.6; $p = 0.03$), aortic arch (cancer = 6.8 ± 2.6; healthy = 5.7 ± 1.9; $p = 0.04$), and descending aorta (cancer = 7.5 ± 3.0; healthy = 6.1 ± 1.7; $p = 0.02$). In addition, patients with angina pectoris were observed with higher TBR in the aortic arch compared with that of healthy subjects (angina = 6.9 ± 3.0; healthy = 5.7 ± 1.9; $p = 0.04$).

After adjusting for age and sex, a significant increase in TBR was observed in patients with prostate cancer compared with healthy controls at the ascending aorta ($p = 0.04$), aortic arch ($p = 0.03$), and descending aorta ($p = 0.04$). Age- and sex-adjusted comparisons between healthy subjects and patients with angina pectoris revealed significant differences at the ascending aorta ($p = 0.03$) and aortic arch ($p = 0.04$) (**Table 1**). No significant differences in TBR were oberved between prostate cancer patients and angina pectoris patients in the coronary arteries or any segment of the aorta with or without multivariable adjustment.

DISCUSSION

To the best of our knowledge, this is the first study to examine aortic and coronary artery NaF uptake in patients with prostate cancer. In this study, NaF uptake in the coronary arteries, aortic arch, ascending aorta, and descending aorta were all observed to be significantly greater in patients with cancer than in healthy controls. These results support the feasibility of using NaF-PET/CT to assess active vascular microcalcification because of atherosclerosis.

Cancer and cardiovascular disease are two leading causes of morbidity worldwide, and these disease processes have been found to share common molecular and mechanical pathways, including oxidative stress and angiogenesis.[3,42] Suzuki and colleagues[43] found that 1020 day incidence of cancers (5% vs 2%, $p = 0.0001$) and overall mortality (6% vs 3%, $p = 0.0001$) was significantly increased in 10,592 patients with atherosclerosis compared with 21,503 non-atherosclerotic patients. Neugut and colleagues[44]

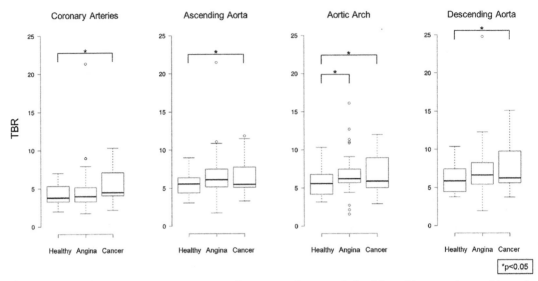

Fig. 1. Box-and-whisker plots showing NaF uptake expressed as TBRs in healthy subjects, patients with angina pectoris, and patients with prostate cancer in the coronary arteries, ascending aorta, aortic arch, and descending aorta.

meanwhile observed that prostate cancer, but not breast or colorectal cancers, is associated with a significantly increased risk of coronary artery disease. Collectively, these studies implicate cardiovascular disease as a major source of comorbidity in patients with cancer.

Atherosclerosis has traditionally been diagnosed by structural changes, including virtual histology intravascular ultrasound, X-ray angiography, and CT.[45] Over the past two decades, inflammation has become a target for research and therapy of atherosclerotic disease.[46] FDG-PET/CT, a sensitive and specific imaging modality in inflammatory processes, is a feasible imaging modality to visualize atherosclerotic vasculitis. Yun and colleagues[47] studied 156 patients (130 controls, 26 patients diagnosed with coronary artery disease) and observed that subjects with coronary artery disease showed significantly increased FDG uptake in the iliac artery and the proximal femoral artery. However, the same study noted that over 50% of the study sample, regardless of cardiovascular disease status, showed some level of arterial FDG, and FDG uptake within the abdominal aorta was not different between the groups.

The ability of FDG-PET/CT to differentiate between inflammatory and non-inflammatory atherosclerotic plaques has been brought into question by Dilsizian and Jadvar.[48] On the contrary, NaF-PET/CT has recently shown promise in the detection and quantification of atherosclerosis. Derlin and colleagues[49] show that NaF-PET/CT is a feasible modality to measure mineral depositions

Table 1
Target-to-background ratios of healthy subjects, patients with angina pectoris, and patients with prostate cancer in the coronary arteries, ascending aorta, aortic arch, and descending aorta

Vessel	Healthy Subjects (TBR)	Patients with angina pectoris (TBR)	Patients with prostate cancer (TBR)	Healthy vs Angina (Age- and Sex-Adjusted p-value)	Healthy vs Cancer (Age- and Sex-Adjusted p-value)
Coronary arteries	4.2 ± 1.4	4.9 ± 3.4	5.3 ± 2.1	0.21	0.15
Ascending aorta	5.4 ± 1.6	6.7 ± 3.5	6.6 ± 2.4	0.03	0.04
Aortic arch	5.7 ± 1.9	6.9 ± 3.0	6.8 ± 2.6	0.04	0.03
Descending aorta	6.1 ± 1.7	7.2 ± 3.9	7.5 ± 3.0	0.07	0.04

of atherosclerosis. Blomberg and colleagues[7,40] observed that both aortic and coronary calcifications measured by NaF-PET/CT are significantly increased with increasing risk of cardiovascular disease. Moreover, Arani and colleagues[50] found that NaF uptake, but not FDG uptake, within the abdominal aorta is significantly associated with 10-year Framingham Risk Score for cardiovascular disease. Paydary and colleagues[51] meanwhile implicated increased thoracic aortic uptake of NaF with cardiovascular disease risk. Taken together, the aorta and carotid arteries may represent strong candidates for global quantification by NaF-PET/CT. This study further shows the value of NaF-PET/CT to detect vascular calcification.

Our results should be interpreted within the confines of our study design. We found significantly higher NaF uptake in patients with cancer compared to healthy subjects. It might be argued that the use of different PET/CT systems might influence the results. However, there were not significant differences in uptake between patients with cancer and patients with angina pectoris, making a systematic inequitable distribution less likely. TBR measurements further minimized the variability of scanner performance and therefore the data generated for this study. In addition, a number of confounding variables, such as medications and differences in age and sex between the three groups, were not accounted for in our analysis. Increased average age in the cancer group in particular may confound the effect caused by cancer. Regarding future research, we believe that large prospective studies will help characterize the link between cancer and atherosclerotic change quantified by NaF-PET/CT.

In summary, our global quantitative assessment showed a significant increase in arterial wall NaF uptake in patients with cancer compared with healthy subjects, suggestive of the presence of increased ongoing arterial calcification. Future prospective studies with a larger number of subjects are necessary to further validate this interesting observation, which may prove valuable in the management of patients with cancer with comorbid atherosclerosis.

SUMMARY

NaF-PET/CT reveals increased vascular microcalcification in the coronary arteries and aorta of patients with prostate cancer compared with healthy control subjects and a similar degree of microcalcification to that of patients with angina pectoris and therefore may serve as a useful marker for comorbid atherosclerosis in cancer.

CLINICS CARE POINTS

- Recent studies suggest that NaF activity is better correlated with cardiovascular risk factors compared to FDG and therefore may become the PET tracer of choice for atherosclerosis imaging.

- The results of the present study show that angina pectoris and prostate cancer are both associated with increased NaF avidity at the aortic arch compared to healthy controls, confirming the sensitivity of this technique to detect expected differences between patient populations.

- NaF-PET/CT was further able to demonstrate increased microcalcification of the coronary arteries in prostate cancer patients compared to healthy controls. Therefore, the assessment of coronary artery disease is a feasible and clinically relevant application of NaF-PET/CT that is impossible with FDG-PET/CT due to physiologic myocardial activity of the latter.

FUNDING

This research received no external funding.

INSTITUTIONAL REVIEW BOARD STATEMENT

The study was conducted in accordance with the Declaration of Helsinki and approved by the Institutional Review Board of the University of Pennsylvania (protocol # 806,020, approved on June 15, 2016).

INFORMED CONSENT STATEMENT

Patient consent was waived due to the retrospective nature of this study, which presented no more than minimal risk to its subjects.

CONFLICTS OF INTEREST

The authors declare no conflict of interest.

REFERENCES

1. Benjamin EJ, Muntner P, Alonso A, et al. Heart disease and stroke statistics-2019 update: a report from the american heart association. Circulation 2019;139:e56–528.

2. McMillan DE. Blood flow and the localization of atherosclerotic plaques. Stroke 1985;16:582–7.

3. Tapia-Vieyra JV, Delgado-Coello B, Mas-Oliva J. Atherosclerosis and cancer; a resemblance with far-reaching implications. Arch Med Res 2017;48: 12–26.

4. Ross JS, Stagliano NE, Donovan MJ, et al. Atherosclerosis and cancer: common molecular pathways of disease development and progression. Ann N Y Acad Sci 2001;947:271–92 [discussion: 292-273].

5. Steinl DC, Kaufmann BA. Ultrasound imaging for risk assessment in atherosclerosis. Int J Mol Sci 2015; 16:9749–69.

6. Kramer CM, Anderson JD. MRI of atherosclerosis: diagnosis and monitoring therapy. Expert Rev Cardiovasc Ther 2007;5:69–80.

7. Blomberg BA, de Jong PA, Thomassen A, et al. Thoracic aorta calcification but not inflammation is associated with increased cardiovascular disease risk: results of the CAMONA study. Eur J Nucl Med Mol Imaging 2017;44:249–58.

8. Irkle A, Vesey AT, Lewis DY, et al. Identifying active vascular microcalcification by (18)F-sodium fluoride positron emission tomography. Nat Commun 2015; 6:7495.

9. Fonager RF, Zacho HD, Langkilde NC, et al. Diagnostic test accuracy study of (18)F-sodium fluoride PET/CT, (99m)Tc-labelled diphosphonate SPECT/CT, and planar bone scintigraphy for diagnosis of bone metastases in newly diagnosed, high-risk prostate cancer. Am J Nucl Med Mol Imaging 2017;7:218–27.

10. Fiz F, Morbelli S, Piccardo A, et al. 1)(8)F-NaF uptake by atherosclerotic plaque on PET/CT imaging: inverse correlation between calcification density and mineral metabolic activity. J Nucl Med 2015; 56:1019–23.

11. Mick CG, James T, Hill JD, et al. Molecular imaging in oncology: (18)F-sodium fluoride PET imaging of osseous metastatic disease. AJR Am J Roentgenol 2014;203:263–71.

12. Al-Zaghal A, Aras M, Borja AJ, et al. Detection of pulmonary artery atherosclerosis by FDG-PET/CT: a new observation. Am J Nucl Med Mol Imaging 2020;10:127–34.

13. Alavi A, Werner TJ, Raynor W, et al. Critical review of PET imaging for detection and characterization of the atherosclerotic plaques with emphasis on limitations of FDG-PET compared to NaF-PET in this setting. Am J Nucl Med Mol Imaging 2021;11: 337–51.

14. Arani LS, Zirakchian Zadeh M, Saboury B, et al. Assessment of atherosclerosis in multiple myeloma and smoldering myeloma patients using (18)F- sodium fluoride PET/CT. J Nucl Cardiol 2021;28: 3044–54.

15. Asadollahi S, Rojulpote C, Bhattaru A, et al. Comparison of atherosclerotic burden in non-lower extremity arteries in patients with and without peripheral artery disease using (18)F-NaF-PET/CT imaging. Am J Nucl Med Mol Imaging 2020;10:272–8.

16. Bhattaru A, Rojulpote C, Gonuguntla K, et al. An understanding of the atherosclerotic molecular calcific heterogeneity between coronary, upper limb, abdominal, and lower extremity arteries as assessed by NaF PET/CT. Am J Nucl Med Mol Imaging 2021; 11:40–5.

17. Blomberg BA, Thomassen A, de Jong PA, et al. Impact of personal characteristics and technical factors on quantification of sodium 18F-Fluoride uptake in human arteries: prospective evaluation of healthy subjects. J Nucl Med 2015;56:1534–40.

18. Borja AJ, Bhattaru A, Rojulpote C, et al. Association between atherosclerotic cardiovascular disease risk score estimated by pooled cohort equation and coronary plaque burden as assessed by NaF-PET/CT. Am J Nucl Med Mol Imaging 2020;10:312–8.

19. Borja AJ, Rojulpote C, Hancin EC, et al. An update on the role of total-body PET imaging in the evaluation of atherosclerosis. PET Clin 2020;15:477–85.

20. Brodsky L, Chesnais H, Piri R, et al. Association of baseline subject characteristics with changes in coronary calcification assessed by (18)F-sodium fluoride PET/CT. Hell J Nucl Med 2021;24:45–52.

21. Castro SA, Muser D, Lee H, et al. Carotid artery molecular calcification assessed by [(18)F]fluoride PET/CT: correlation with cardiovascular and thromboembolic risk factors. Eur Radiol 2021;31:8050–9.

22. Gonuguntla K, Rojulpote C, Patil S, et al. Utilization of NaF-PET/CT in assessing global cardiovascular calcification using CHADS2 and CHADS2-VASc scoring systems in high risk individuals for cardiovascular disease. Am J Nucl Med Mol Imaging 2020;10:293–300.

23. Hancin EC, Raynor WY, Borja AJ, et al. Non-(18)F-FDG/(18)F-NaF radiotracers proposed for the diagnosis and management of diseases of the heart and vasculature. PET Clin 2021;16:273–84.

24. Hoilund-Carlsen PF, Piri R, Constantinescu C, et al. Atherosclerosis imaging with (18)F-sodium fluoride PET. Diagnostics (Basel) 2020;10.

25. Hoilund-Carlsen PF, Sturek M, Alavi A, et al. Atherosclerosis imaging with (18)F-sodium fluoride PET: state-of-the-art review. Eur J Nucl Med Mol Imaging 2020;47:1538–51.

26. Koa B, Borja AJ, Yellanki D, et al. 18)F-FDG-PET/CT in the assessment of atherosclerosis in lung cancer. Am J Nucl Med Mol Imaging 2021;11:1–9.

27. Mayer M, Borja AJ, Hancin EC, et al. Imaging atherosclerosis by PET, with emphasis on the role of FDG and NaF as potential biomarkers for this disorder. Front Physiol 2020;11:511391.

28. McKenney-Drake ML, Moghbel MC, Paydary K, et al. 18)F-NaF and (18)F-FDG as molecular probes in the evaluation of atherosclerosis. Eur J Nucl Med Mol Imaging 2018;45:2190–200.

29. Patil S, Rojulpote C, Gonuguntla K, et al. Association of triglyceride to high density lipoprotein ratio with global cardiac microcalcification to evaluate subclinical coronary atherosclerosis in non-diabetic individuals. Am J Cardiovasc Dis 2020;10:241–6.

30. Paydary K, Revheim ME, Emamzadehfard S, et al. Quantitative thoracic aorta calcification assessment by (18)F-NaF PET/CT and its correlation with atherosclerotic cardiovascular disorders and increasing age. Eur Radiol 2021;31:785–94.

31. Raynor WY, Borja AJ, Rojulpote C, et al. (18)F-sodium fluoride: an emerging tracer to assess active vascular microcalcification. J Nucl Cardiol 2021;28: 2706–11.

32. Raynor WY, Park PSU, Borja AJ, et al. PET-based imaging with (18)F-FDG and (18)F-NaF to assess inflammation and microcalcification in atherosclerosis and other vascular and thrombotic disorders. Diagnostics (Basel) 2021;11.

33. Rojulpote C, Borja AJ, Zhang V, et al. Role of (18)F-NaF-PET in assessing aortic valve calcification with age. Am J Nucl Med Mol Imaging 2020;10:47–56.

34. Rojulpote C, Patil S, Gonuguntla K, et al. NaF-PET/CT global assessment in detecting and quantifying subclinical cardiac atherosclerosis and its association with blood pressure in non-dyslipidemic individuals. Am J Cardiovasc Dis 2020;10:101–7.

35. Saboury B, Edenbrandt L, Piri R, et al. Alavi-carlsen calcification score (ACCS): a Simple measure of global cardiac atherosclerosis burden. Diagnostics (Basel) 2021;11:1421.

36. Seraj SM, Raynor WY, Revheim ME, et al. Assessing the feasibility of NaF-PET/CT versus FDG-PET/CT to detect abdominal aortic calcification or inflammation in rheumatoid arthritis patients. Ann Nucl Med 2020; 34:424–31.

37. Sorci O, Batzdorf AS, Mayer M, et al. 18)F-sodium fluoride PET/CT provides prognostic clarity compared to calcium and Framingham risk scoring when addressing whole-heart arterial calcification. Eur J Nucl Med Mol Imaging 2020;47:1678–87.

38. Zhang V, Borja AJ, Rojulpote C, et al. Global quantification of pulmonary artery atherosclerosis using (18)F-sodium fluoride PET/CT in at-risk subjects. Am J Nucl Med Mol Imaging 2020;10:119–26.

39. Beheshti M, Mottaghy FM, Paycha F, et al. 18)F-NaF PET/CT: EANM procedure guidelines for bone imaging. Eur J Nucl Med Mol Imaging 2015; 42:1767–77.

40. Blomberg BA, Thomassen A, de Jong PA, et al. Coronary fluorine-18-sodium fluoride uptake is increased in healthy adults with an unfavorable cardiovascular risk profile: results from the CAMONA study. Nucl Med Commun 2017;38:1007–14.

41. Raynor W, Ayubcha C, Pourhassan Shamchi S, et al. Assessing global uptake of 18F-sodium fluoride in the femoral neck: a novel quantitative technique to evaluate changes in bone turnover with age. J Nucl Med 2017;58:1223.

42. Sies H. Oxidative stress: oxidants and antioxidants. Exp Physiol 1997;82:291–5.

43. Suzuki M, Tomoike H, Sumiyoshi T, et al. Incidence of cancers in patients with atherosclerotic cardiovascular diseases. Int J Cardiol Heart Vasc 2017;17: 11–6.

44. Neugut AI, Rosenberg DJ, Ahsan H, et al. Association between coronary heart disease and cancers of the breast, prostate, and colon. Cancer Epidemiol Biomarkers Prev 1998;7:869–73.

45. Tarkin JM, Dweck MR, Evans NR, et al. Imaging atherosclerosis. Circ Res 2016;118:750–69.

46. Li B, Li W, Li X, et al. Inflammation: a novel therapeutic target/direction in atherosclerosis. Curr Pharm Des 2017;23:1216–27.

47. Yun M, Jang S, Cucchiara A, et al. 18F FDG uptake in the large arteries: a correlation study with the atherogenic risk factors. Semin Nucl Med 2002;32: 70–6.

48. Dilsizian V, Jadvar H. Science to practice: does FDG differentiate morphologically unstable from stable atherosclerotic plaque? Radiology 2017;283:1–3.

49. Derlin T, Richter U, Bannas P, et al. Feasibility of 18F-sodium fluoride PET/CT for imaging of atherosclerotic plaque. J Nucl Med 2010;51:862–5.

50. Arani LS, Gharavi MH, Zadeh MZ, et al. Association between age, uptake of (18)F-fluorodeoxyglucose and of (18)F-sodium fluoride, as cardiovascular risk factors in the abdominal aorta. Hell J Nucl Med 2019;22:14–9.

51. Paydary K, Emamzadehfard S, Gholami S, et al. 18F-NaF PET/CT quantification of vascular calcification in the thoracic aorta is associated with increasing age and presence of cardiovascular risk factors. J Nucl Med 2017;58:298.

Printed and bound by CPI Group (UK) Ltd, Croydon, CR0 4YY

03/10/2024

01040307-0008